JOANNA THOMSON was born a~~~~~~~~ Kingston Nature
Cure Clinic. The Clinic in Edinburgh was ~~~~~~~ d in 1918 by her

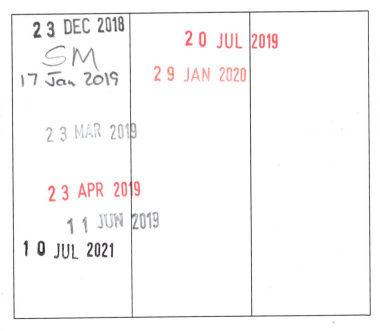

Live Well.
Eat Well.
Be Well.

A Guide to Natural and Healthy Living

JOANNA THOMSON

Luath Press Limited
EDINBURGH
www.luath.co.uk

First published 2017
New updated edition 2018

ISBN: 978-1-912147-40-3

The paper used in this book is recyclable. It is made from
low chlorine pulps produced in a low energy, low emissions manner
from renewable forests.

Printed and bound by
Bell & Bain Ltd., Glasgow

Typeset in 10 point Sabon by
3btype.com

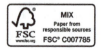

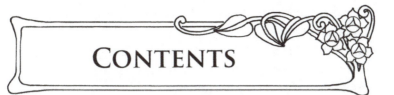

CONTENTS

ACKNOWLEDGEMENTS

I would like to thank the Tait Vision Fund for their support, my family for being different from the norm on both sides and for fighting all the battles so that I didn't have to. I would like to give credit to all the Kingston trained Nature Cure practitioners and those following the lifestyle who have all added something along the way. I would also like to thank Jan, Jean and Lesley for being a supportive critic, flying the flag and prodding me when I got bogged down, respectively.

But mostly I'd like to thank my two sons Alan and Martin for being healthy, happy and communicative and finally Rosie and Sweet Pea, my two highland ponies for making me go outside whatever the weather and for keeping me sane.

All royalties derived from the sale of this book will be donated to the Tait Vision Fund.

Joanna Thomson

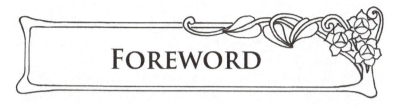

FOREWORD

IN JULY 2013, having finished writing a book on the future of Scotland, I was exhausted. Not the usual kind of brain-dead lethargy that sets in after too many early mornings, late nights and prolonged sessions at the laptop but a real, deep-seated inability to get going or rouse myself to do anything. I'm no athlete but I always used to perk up at the prospect of getting outdoors on a bike or up a glen during the long days of summer. Suddenly neither prospect appealed. Even two weeks in North Uist on the Outer Hebrides – mostly writing of course – had failed to work its usual magic. I was, to use the parlance, knackered.

Passing through Ullapool on the way home, I stopped off to see my good friend, Jean Urquhart, MSP and proprietor of the Ceilidh Place. She sat me down, brewed some herbal tea – most emphatically not coffee – and started to explain Naturopathy. It seemed Jean had been using 'Nature Cure' for several decades – with occasional tumbles 'off the wagon.' My curiosity built. Flicking through the well-thumbed booklets on her shelf, I began to realise I had no idea how my body worked or what I really needed to stay healthy. I'd been running at full tilt for decades, piling on pressure, using coffee to stay awake, eating whatever came to hand and burning the candle at both ends – in other words, a fairly typical modern Scotswoman. But finally I was getting curious about living differently.

It was a genuinely life-changing moment.

Once home, I sought out Joanna Thomson – the daughter of the man who had so impressed Jean Urquhart a few decades earlier. Like father, like daughter.

I stopped using salt, coffee, tea, lemon, vinegar and painkillers. Started eating fresh fruit for breakfast, first thing every day. Planted lettuce, ate salad and stopped eating processed food. There are still pizzas in the deep freeze that pre-date this big change. Within four weeks I stopped having a slight wheeze and sinus problems. I grew long fingernails (despite typing) that were almost bulletproof for the first time in my life. I felt pretty good. Just as well.

A few weeks later at hospital in Kirkcaldy I was diagnosed with a potentially serious auto-immune condition, given a kidney biopsy and put on chemotherapy. Perhaps if I had been an apprentice Naturopath longer I might have thought twice about the treatment. But I went ahead – and concentrated on being the best, healthiest patient I could be. Mercifully, it seems to have worked thus far.

I realise the placebo effect is powerful. I understand there are many other dietary regimes. But Nature Cure makes sense to me, costs nothing and puts a premium on eating nutrition packed, home grown vegetables not empty, factory-made food.

It's an outlook I could usefully have stumbled over a little earlier in life. And I'm delighted Joanna is making sure no future generation has that excuse.

Lesley Riddoch

PREFACE

THIS BOOK IS THE distillation, and a much abridged version, of the work of three generations of Nature Cure practitioners; James C Thomson, Jessie R Thomson and C Leslie Thomson – my grandfather, grandmother and father respectively – all of whom were published authors. But this is much, much more than a collection of historic writings, because, although this pioneering group established Nature Cure in Scotland back in the early 20th century, so much of what they wrote then is still pertinent today.

My grandfather, James C Thomson, was blunt, rude and a trailblazer. He had to be right; he had to believe that he was always right. Fortunately, he very often was. My grandmother, Jessie, followed quietly and graciously in his wake, unruffling feathers and being a very effective practitioner in her own right. My father, Leslie, was a talented amateur electronics engineer, photographer and author, but he was also a brilliant naturopath. His approach tended to be more mechanistic but he always acknowledged the emotional aspects of his patients' problems and this made him a perfect co-director at the Kingston Clinic to my uncle Sandy. Alec (Sandy) Milne's approach tended to have more emphasis on the psycho (of the mind) before the somatic (of the body). These four naturopaths have left a wonderful heritage of monographs and books, but they needed to be updated and edited. This book draws on the work of my family, both written and remembered. *Live Well. Eat Well. Be Well.* is intended to be a day-to-day handbook for those in need of a lifestyle change to regain, and thereafter maintain, their health.

The book covers a wide range of conditions and offers common sense solutions and advice for self-help and home treatments. The original works were written in a rather paternalistic tone, which was fine 50 years ago but goes over less well in 2016, so some revising and updating was required. However, the methodologies, information and advice of the Nature Cure have changed remarkably little in over 100 years, so it only needed to be presented in a more approachable style. The original wisdom and knowledge is still there, and as fresh and applicable today as ever. I did, at times, struggle with having to so severely edit my forebears' work, often feeling like they were looking over my shoulder as I wrote, but there was a need for a fresh overview from the third generation. After all, this is good stuff and should be out there. Some passages have changed very little from the original – the message is clear and unambiguous.

The exciting thing is that although the beginnings of 'modern' Nature Cure date back well over two centuries it is still absolutely right for today. It is in tune with the need to take less from our shared planet, it chimes with the growing interest in where our food comes from, it concurs with the need to find a path to health other than via pharmaceuticals and it corresponds with the urgent need to seriously re-adjust what is currently the orthodox approach to health. And it's been there all along – it's just been a bit lost behind the clamour about the next exciting super food.

The more I researched, the more I found recent studies that underpinned what we had been teaching for years and years. Too often things that are heralded as amazing new discoveries are what we have been teaching for decades. You will find that some chapters have references, while others do not. This is because the ones without the references *were* the original research papers, the evidence of efficacy, based on 50 years of residential practice.

So, this book will help you to live more healthily and get more out of life without it costing the earth, or you a fortune. You will also discover ways to take control of your own health. Nature Cure is a way of life that is affordable, straightforward and very empowering. I know it is, because I live it, and when I don't my body soon lets me know!

I asked J S, a long-standing Kingstonite, for her experience with the Kingston Nature Cure:

> I have been a follower of Kingston Nature Cure since I was a baby, 78 years ago. My mother could not afford to pay so we saw the students, who were supervised by Miss Atkinson.
>
> We were brought up the Kingston way – no medicine, no vaccinations and cold compresses when necessary. At school all vaccinations were refused and the doctor there said we were being neglected. As a result of this my mother had to go and report to the medical referee for health in Edinburgh. She explained why and told him about Kingston. To my mother's surprise he told her that no one had told him she went to Kingston. From now on, he said, she would have no problems with school doctors!

INTRODUCTION

ARE YOU FED UP reading about the 'latest health cure' in the popular press? Have you lost faith in miracle drugs that don't produce the promised outcomes? Have you become a little skeptical about the latest proclaimed super food? Are you looking for something well established, tried and tested, that actually works and better yet, doesn't involve any pharmaceuticals? Are you prepared to put in some real effort to improve your health?

Every generation thinks that they have found all the answers, and too often their claims are ridiculed by the next. But there is a lifestyle choice that is over 200 years old and is still effective and straightforward and has no gimmicks or unpleasant side effects. This is Natural Therapeutics or Nature Cure.

If you are new to Nature Cure the adjustments we will ask you to make to your lifestyle might initially prove to be rather challenging and more than a little daunting. They might appear to be too unconventional, too different from the norm. But if you can stick with it you will find that your new ways of living are really very basic and honest. We understand that changing your habits is difficult; we accept that it means leaving your comfort zone and being prepared to question the status quo.

You could look at it the same way as upgrading your computer or phone. It can be annoying and troublesome to learn the new systems, the buttons are broadly the same but the functions have changed subtly. You persevere and almost magically, with a little time, things are made easier, more fun and more flexible.

Living the Nature Cure life means being allowed and enabled

to take a lot more responsibility for your own health, possibly for the first time. According to recent research only some 10 per cent of people in the UK take that responsibility, the other 90 per cent apparently being content to hand this duty over to their local health service. Nature Cure encourages you to ask questions and to do your own research and this book gives you some of the tools you need to make a start. We understand that changing habits can be scary, but it can also be both empowering and life affirming.

To follow Nature Cure means accepting that ill health rarely, if ever, happens without a reason, and there will always be cause and effect at work. The information and advice in this book is based on a century of observations in outpatient and residential practice by one extended family and is presented with a liberal dose of simple, good old common sense.

As James C Thomson put it nearly a century ago:

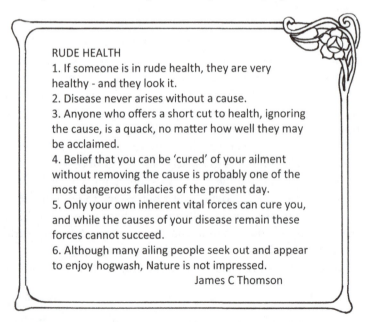

RUDE HEALTH
1. If someone is in rude health, they are very healthy - and they look it.
2. Disease never arises without a cause.
3. Anyone who offers a short cut to health, ignoring the cause, is a quack, no matter how well they may be acclaimed.
4. Belief that you can be 'cured' of your ailment without removing the cause is probably one of the most dangerous fallacies of the present day.
5. Only your own inherent vital forces can cure you, and while the causes of your disease remain these forces cannot succeed.
6. Although many ailing people seek out and appear to enjoy hogwash, Nature is not impressed.
James C Thomson

Global Health Crisis

We are reaching a crisis point in many areas of the human condition and not least in medical science. In the summer of 2013 The Chief Medical Officer for England, Professor Dame Sally Davies, announced that antibiotics resistance is 'as big a risk as terrorism'. In her book *The Drugs Don't Work*[1] she calls for new drugs to be developed by the pharmaceutical companies. In effect, Dame Sally would like to see more of the same thing that created the problem in the first place. Yet she also warns that we need to address our relationship with antimicrobials and goes on to paint an apocalyptic scenario, in which people will again die from routine infections.

Microbes

There is no quibble that viruses and bacterial organisms are out there, but they are also inside us – our alimentary tract is full of 'helpful' bacteria (weighing, in total, between 2–3kg in a healthy individual) and our skin has a fair population of them too – and it is also true that 'bad' bacteria and viruses 'invade' our bodies from time to time. Bacteria are around us all the time and every now and then a particular strain will start to dominate, but no matter how virulent they are, not everyone has the same response.

Our bodies are amazing self-regulating, self-repairing organisms. They are endowed with an incredible somatic intelligence and too often we try to override that intelligence by employing hugely toxic substances to suppress symptoms of disease. We blithely assume that our conscious (learned) intelligence has some superior knowledge of the situation. But as we attempt to suppress the

---

1   Davies, Professor Dame Sally. *The Drugs Don't Work*. Penguin Special. September 2013

uncomfortable symptoms we are also taking the commonly held erroneous view that we somehow 'know better' than our body. Our bodies, those amazing organisms that regulate the growth of a baby from conception to birth, all without any conscious interference by the mother. Our bodies, that can knit broken bones without our help (yes, it's true that a skilled surgeon is needed to set broken bones, but thereafter it is the body that does the healing). Our bodies, that can adapt to all sorts of situations and environments, that regulate our heartbeat, cell replacement and a million other activities without any 'helpful' interference from our conscious minds.

Symptoms

Are you interested in listening to your body and working with its natural healing capabilities? Have you started to realise that treating the symptoms of illness has often brought you back to where you started, after only a temporary respite? Are you having nagging doubts that taking suppressive medicines is not the right way forward? Would you rather investigate the causes of your ailment and get to the root of the problem? Then read on.

So what do we have to offer to someone looking for a genuine alternative to medicine? We have no magic pills, no clever liquids in bottles, no creams, no lotions and no potions to sell. We have no gimmicks, nothing that you can take away in a pretty bag and administer to yourself. So what do we believe in?

In a nutshell, Nature Cure is all about a straightforward way of life; a whole way of life. The approach embraces and informs all aspects of your lifestyle, it teaches the importance of honest nutrition, believes that fresh air, exercise and sleep are vital to good health. Nature Cure accepts that your emotional life and your home and work environment are vitally important. It also uses water therapies to assist the body's natural healing activities. Nature Cure does not promise to be a panacea, however we are here to guide you in a different way of living and to help you to look at your life – and illnesses – afresh. We do not claim to have all the answers, but then nobody does. We do have some excellent suggestions and advice and sound methods and many, many years of clinical experience to draw on.

In the words of C Leslie Thomson from 1975:

> Thomson Kingston Nature Cure is not, and makes no pretence to be, a substitute for medication. It cannot be produced in doses for specific ailments, and although this may sound strange, it is not primarily a resort for people when they are ill. It is much bigger than that. Naturopathy is a way of life and a way of looking at life, and a way of applying reasoned interpretation to what is observed.

Alec Milne, on the other hand, considered that it is only in Nature Cure that there is a philosophical alternative to medicine, where the symptom is seen as a signpost to be followed and a condition to be understood, rather than an enemy to be defeated or quashed. It is essentially an all-inclusive approach to health and we really prefer it to be preventative. Nature Cure means what it says: that cure is to be sought by reaching back to nature; by recognising that the curative power is the *vis Medicatrix Naturae*, the Healing Power of Nature — (ironically the motto of the medical profession). The essential role of a Nature Cure practitioner is to create a situation where the individual gains the confidence to listen to their body's somatic intelligence and to trust the body's innate healing capabilities.

Chapters

Your body is not a collection of spare parts randomly put together, it is a finely tuned organism, an integrated whole. In much the same way that an active and self-sustaining community has resilience to shocks and changes, the body that is seen as a whole integrated organism, and is treated with respect, will withstand life's knocks so much better. Although we Naturopaths don't compartmentalise disease, for the sake of simplicity and to assist you to find the information you feel most relevant to you, this book is divided into chapters that sometimes relate to different parts of the body. As you read through the chapters you will see themes emerging. Even though the title of the chapter may refer to one particular organ, or group of organs, be under no illusions, if one part of your body is distressed then the whole organism is distressed. If you are sceptical about this aspect of our philosophy just think how difficult it is to concentrate on a task while you are suffering from toothache or a sore stomach.

Finally

So often it's not what you add it's what you take away. Medicating, suppressing or masking the negative effects of harmful habits does not add up to a genuine cure. You need to pay heed to the causes, and address these, before real health can be achieved.

LIVE WELL. EAT WELL. BE WELL.

PART ONE

This section lays the foundation stones. It explains our approach, methods and philosophy. It also illustrates why attention to every part of your life, and your lifestyle choices, is important to achieving a healthy life.

All the different aspects combine to build the complete picture, in that way life is a little like the simple nine-piece jigsaw below. Of course you can still function without all the parts – and most of us have to at different times in our lives – but for really good health each aspect should be valued as much as any other.

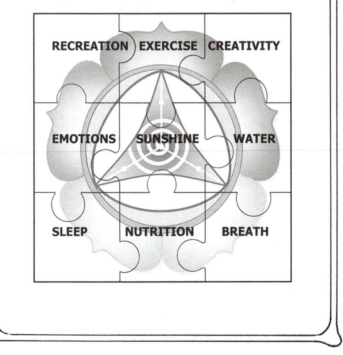

RECREATION EXERCISE CREATIVITY

EMOTIONS SUNSHINE WATER

SLEEP NUTRITION BREATH

CHAPTER ONE
THE NATURE CURE APPROACH

The philosophy and science of nature cure

NATURE CURE IS NOT, and makes no pretence to be, a substitute for medication. It is not primarily a resort for people when they are ill. It is much bigger than that. Nature Cure is a way of life and a way of looking at life, a way of applying reasoned interpretation to what is observed. By doing this, if you accept and practise Nature Cure's philosophy, you too can give your body a better chance of maintaining normal function, or of regaining function when it has been lost. And, as with any worthwhile way of life, Nature Cure is not merely for high days and holidays but for every day.

A philosophical attitude to life, health and illness is an essential feature of the Nature Cure way of life, and our methods are logical, science based, well researched and tried and tested. We believe that illness, and the pain that generally accompanies illness, is no accident and it always has rational causes, so it is important that there is an understanding of illness processes. Bacteria and viruses are interesting and complicating factors in many conditions, but they are generally influenced by the pre-existing condition of the tissues of the body.

Our understanding is based on the same anatomy and physiology as any other medical model, but it is our interpretation of the information that so often differs. For us the physical aspects alone are not enough; your emotions and your mental state are every bit as important to good health as your diet, exercise choices or sleep routines. Your posture, and its effect on your musculo-skeletal structure is an important factor and offer us useful feedback on your overall state of health. Our Nature Cure approach has evolved through decades of observation and the application of simple therapeutic methods.

So, although we are less interested in a diagnosis of a particular illness-with-a-name, what we have done for the last 100 years or so could certainly be described as 'evidence based'.[1] And this is very much something that is called into question by the critics of other alternative health approaches.

---

1 Evidence Based Medicine.

According to the British Medical Journal Volume 312 January 1996:

Evidence based medicine is the conscientious, explicit, and judicious use of current best evidence in making decisions about the care of individual patients. The practice of evidence based medicine means integrating individual clinical expertise with the best available external clinical evidence from systematic research*.

By individual clinical expertise we mean the proficiency and judgement that individual clinicians acquire through clinical experience and clinical practice.

Increased expertise is reflected in many ways, but especially in more effective and efficient diagnosis and in the more thoughtful identification and compassionate use of individual patients' predicaments, rights, and the preferences in making clinical decisions about their care.

As Nature Cure practitioners we have always actively studied good health, rather than pathology, for the answers and this sets us apart from many of the traditional medical models, we also ask 'why has the individual become ill?' We seek the causes of the disease.

So what makes our methods different? This can be illustrated by considering, for instance, someone who has a persistent headache and seeks some relief. They may consult a variety of orthodox or alternative practitioners about their problem; the first might prescribe an analgesic, perhaps combined with an anti-depressant. Another could offer to sell them herbal remedies, but essentially intend to have the same effects as the orthodox prescription. Still other advisers would propose to make them less aware of their distress, perhaps through hypnotism, or by some form of mental exercise or by suggestion.

On principle, the Nature Cure approach rejects all of the above methods. There is no doubt that all of them work in the short term, but the one thing they all have in common is that they are making no attempt to understand or to rectify the *causes* of the discomfort. Each one is treating the symptoms, the illness; they are not treating the whole person. The Nature Cure philosophy demands that before applying even so apparently obvious a remedy as a simple manipulation to relieve the tensions in the neck and shoulders the question must be asked: 'Why does the individual have a headache?'. Headache and neck tension may be due to various primary causes, more often than not a combination of several. But, without seeking to understand at least something about these symptoms and how they came about, it is not possible to give advice or treatment that is likely to be of more than transient benefit.

Symptoms

It is a commonly held belief that a disease is the sum of its symptoms. Although this may seem like a reasonable conclusion, it is also a widespread misconception that is happily and profitably exploited in the sale of every kind of remedy and in encouraging many forms of suppressive symptom treatment. Nature Cure believes that any diseased organism is going to be disordered before the appearance of any symptoms or feelings of discomfort. Most illnesses are quite simply the result of the way we live our lives. If you are properly nourished by a well-balanced wholesome diet; well exercised by a daily brisk walk in the fresh air; rewardingly employed with a reasonable life/work balance; happy in your relationships and emotionally fulfilled; living in an unpolluted environment, then you have an excellent chance of enjoying good health. But even if all these factors are in place there is no guarantee that you can be completely free of illness because there are so many other influences that could undermine your constitution. However, it is possible to say with some confidence that if your life is lacking in one or more of the items on that list, your chance of enjoying good health is reduced. So basically we need to look at all those aspects, and more.

Causes

Our immediate aim is to discover what guidance or advice you might need in such routine matters as diet, exercise, occupational effects, emotional adjustment and the avoidance – as far as possible – of environmental pollutions. That all may sound like common sense today, but despite some enlightenment in orthodox medicine's approach to health, much of the above can still be met with some level of scepticism and a call for scientific proof, or dismissed for lack of some randomised control trial.

We regard acute illnesses as having not only logical causes but also constructive purposes. That is, simple colds, fevers, rashes, sicknesses or diarrhoeas have eliminative or stress-reducing significance. We see them as analogous with spring-cleaning in a household, a time of disturbed routine, of discomfort and commotion, yet with a wholesome and positive purpose. A system that is allowed its occasional 'spring-cleanings' – as necessary to deal with accumulations of waste – has a far better chance of remaining in good working order throughout a long and useful lifetime. But if these unpleasant yet useful processes are promptly arrested by symptomatic treatment – by suppression of the symptoms – the system declines into a state of toxaemia, and the residual accumulations of waste in all the body's tissues results in impaired function. This is the situation in which chronic disease is most likely to develop.

Pain and why it is good to avoid drug treatments

Although us humans usually seek to avoid it, pain serves a very useful purpose; it lets us know that something is wrong. That nagging low backache could be a pointer to over-worked kidneys or a mis-alignment in your lumbar spine and it is only through a thorough consultation that the practitioner can follow the signs to the cause. One big problem is that pain is so often accompanied by fear. Fear of what the pain might mean, what illness the pain might be indicating or fear that the pain might not stop; all these anxieties only serve to amplify your discomfort. If you can do some deep breathing and take stock it's well worth listening to that pain rather than trying to silence it with analgesics, alcohol, recreational or prescription drugs. It is worth taking a closer look at why Nature Cure practitioners don't recommend, 'taking something' for your pain.

We recognise that working towards the root causes of pain can sometimes be very painful in other ways, but it is only once those causes have been identified that positive action can be taken. Following those difficult signposts to the root causes, to the 'why?' of the disruption to your mental and physical health, can be the start of enabling the healing processes to get under way.

There is no doubt that some drug treatments do work, but probably not in the way you would imagine. Many more have dubious outcomes, some are used for conditions they were never developed to treat and a good number of them would not get a license for use if they were new drugs today. They all come with a broad range of side effects, many of which are listed on the labels, but the problem really is that most drugs seem to be developed primarily to make profits for the pharmaceutical companies rather than for the benefit of the sick and unwell. Interestingly, treatments can often be every bit as effective when the patient is given a placebo (a sugar pill) rather than an active substance. Perhaps more so, because in most cases there are no side effects to a sugar pill.

With the placebo effect a large factor in a patient getting better is a change in mental attitude, giving rise to the feeling of hope that can result in a more positive frame of mind. A relaxing of the tensions and fears that have been impeding any progress towards health go a long way to allowing a body to start vital healing processes.

Drugs do not cure; they suppress, mask or alter the symptoms. They do not address the causes of the pre-existing condition that allowed the virus, bacterium, waste storage or debilitating tensions to occur.

Nature Cure encourages you to reach inside yourself for the cure, not for the medicine bottle.

Intrinsic healing

With the Nature Cure approach the real cure will not be instant, but as we all know nothing really worth having is instant. If we are honest with ourselves we will be well aware that it has taken many years of less than helpful daily habits and many different stressors to get to the state of ill health that we find ourselves in. So it follows that it will take a combination of time, acceptance, understanding and effort to move forward to a better state of health in the future. But it will be time and effort well spent. And here it's worth pointing out that time is probably the greatest cost in a Nature Cure lifestyle to achieving good health, all other expenses are minimal.

Fewer antibiotics being prescribed

It might sound like music to a Nature Cure practitioner's ears that, theoretically, fewer prescriptions for antibiotics are being handed out in the doctor's surgery. But let's not get carried away, this is not a shining light from Damascus moment, it is simple expediency on the part of the medical profession. Years of overuse of these drugs by the food industry, and in medicine, means they no longer work as effectively because the bacteria have become more and more resistant to them. Although doctors are now telling patients that self-limiting conditions, like sore throats and even scarlet fever, will get better on their own, there is often a vital link missing. So although we welcome the acceptance by orthodox practitioners that the body can deal with these conditions, there is rarely any reason offered for the disease state arising in the first place or any real credit given to your body's innate healing powers. The simple laws of cause and effect have been at work, but because the National Health Service has historically discouraged us from taking responsibility for our own health, and sometimes even actively dissuaded us from attempting to do so, in the past there had been little effort made to link lifestyle choices to your health. That, at least, is starting to change.

All ages

It may sound like an obvious statement but Nature Cure practitioners prefer to give help and advice to those still in good health. This is not to make the practitioner's life easier, but to enable the individual to maintain good health and realise their true potential. We have much to offer people of all ages and physical fitness; the beneficial effects of proper dietetics upon dentition, general development and muscular endurance are but a few good reasons to establish a healthy way of life as early as possible. However, for people of any age, we also have a useful range of emergency aids, from reduction of pelvic strain, often misdiagnosed as a 'slipped disc', to treatment of injuries, wounds and burns. In the instance of the latter for over 100 years, hydro-therapists have, with outstanding success, treated burns with cold water; a method only now beginning to be partially adopted in orthodox circles. Hydrotherapy methods are, of course, much older than 100 years, and in its current form the therapy has remained relatively unchanged since Vincent Preissnitz (1799–1851) practised in Silesia some 200 years ago.

LIVE WELL. EAT WELL. BE WELL.

Accidental damage or essential surgery

At this point it should be stated that Nature Cure practitioners place high value on surgery in more serious-accident cases or in a case of vital obstruction. However, we have observed that convalescence can be markedly assisted by following simple Nature Cure routines, and in less urgent circumstances there has often been successful co-operation with surgeons, by promoting an improvement in the individual's tissues before the operation, so that healing is rapid, neat and strong. Remember, the surgeon does not do the healing; after the bones are 'set' or the damaged part of the organ removed, the body, and only the body, does the rebuilding and healing work.

It is a sad fact of Nature Cure practice that those who have long been chronically ill, and who have suffered extensive degenerative changes, are likely to turn to our methods as a last resort. Given no hope of future improvement they turn to us for help. Although this could be seen as obliquely flattering, it is an unhappy truth that a true cure in such cases is often not possible. This is because some essential bodily tissues or a part of a vital organ has already been destroyed. Nevertheless, some good, workable recoveries can often be achieved and this is an impressive testimony to the tremendous self-healing powers of the human organism, especially when that healing effort is unopposed and understood. The successful cases are also evidence of understanding and determination on the part of the individual. And there should be no doubt about this; Nature Cure is demanding on the person involved. It calls not only for the effort of accepting routines of treatment and following practices which gradually merge into daily habits, but also for the acceptance of individual responsibility. This latter point is of supreme importance. The foregoing might make it all sound a bit burdensome and difficult, but it really isn't. Nature Cure can actually be remarkably empowering and enjoyable.

No remedies

We must make one thing clear; we do not offer to 'cure' anybody. Our work is essentially educational, with the aim of enabling you to realise your own self-reparative and vital capacities. In the early stages there may need to be some treatments aimed at relieving physical or mental stresses; there will be some advice and guidance that could at times sound quite harsh or we might ask you to do certain things on trust. But until you gain real confidence in your own judgment, and start to believe in the inherent intelligence of your own body, our work is incomplete.

Nature Cure highlights the cumulative detrimental effects of widespread and seemingly innocent daily habits, such as drinking quantities of tea, coffee or soft drinks; all forms of smoking; the consumption of processed foods; the use of 'simple remedies' for constipation, stomach-ache or insomnia and the many other devitalising things we all do in what passes for a normal life. Now, that list might have a familiar ring to it, because these days orthodox medical practitioners have to acknowledge that the way you live your life directly affects your health. But please remember that my grandfather, James C Thomson, was pointing this out a century ago and never stopped saying it. One hundred years later his granddaughter is repeating it.

Our philosophy is very straightforward and we use no remedies, potions or clever devices. We have no place for expensive thermal baths, elixirs, brightly packaged synthetic vitamin concentrates and a whole catalogue of so-called 'health foods' or 'super foods'. Our Nature Cure methods will not involve you in the purchase of such services or merchandise. Our income does not come from profit or commission on sales of remedies, 'health foods' or gadgetry. For many this may be quite disconcerting. Leaving the practice without a bottle or package containing a remedy or supplement leaves you with only one option – to believe in the inherent healing powers within your own body. For most people this means having to trust consciously, for probably the first time in your life, in your own innate somatic intelligence. This is so different from the orthodox approach where the credit for the 'cure' is given to the contents of the bottle or the cleverness of the gadget, not to your amazingly intelligent body.

So what treatments do we offer?

Manipulative therapy is a part of any treatment programme and it can be anything from a simple massage for relaxation to quite strong osteopathic adjustments. It will form an important part of any programme towards good health, but a Nature Cure practitioner does not work mechanically; each case will be individually assessed. Dealing with the causes of a disorder is often more important than giving immediate relief – even though, reasonably enough, you would prefer to get rid of your discomfort as soon as possible. In dietetics, practical information will be included as will the matter of the environment in which you eat. Also as previously mentioned, we draw on a century's worth of practical experience in hydrotherapy supporting our use of simple and effective water applications. Many of which can be safely used in the home in a surprising number of circumstances.

We give equal importance to the psychological significance of symptoms and stresses. We are particularly alert to the ways in which negative emotions may be intensified or diminished by altered physiological states, and how the reverse sequence can occur. Closely linked with psychological influences are problems of poor posture – so often the case with hours spent bent over a computer screen – and this is a broad field in which your emotional and familial background can be every bit as significant as your current occupation.

To quote from an early publication by James C Thomson, one of the founders of The Kingston Clinic, which was established by the Thomson family in 1938 and closed in 1988, having helped hundreds of patients from all over the world to regain their health and embrace a natural, simple and common sense way of life:

> High Level Health is not to be achieved by the efforts of any group of practitioners. There must be intelligent and whole-hearted co-operation by the individual concerned and after it has been achieved it must be just as intelligently sustained by wholesome habits of mind and body.
>
> For this reason, we deliberately avoid any form of treatment which may give dramatic but transient results, and concentrate on those which either can be easily continued at home or will relieve strains for a considerable time after their application.
>
> That is to say, we offer no 'cure' to those who come to Kingston, rather we offer to expound to each individual the causes of his or her illness, and explain how real health can be cultivated.
>
> Kingston, in fact, represents an attitude of mind.

LIVE WELL. EAT WELL. BE WELL.

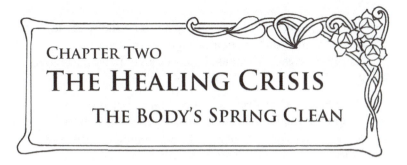

CHAPTER TWO
THE HEALING CRISIS
THE BODY'S SPRING CLEAN

THE HEALING CRISIS is an acute reaction by a normally healthy body to an unhealthy internal condition. It is an effort by nature's positive life force to rid your body of the build-up of toxins *causing* your disease or distressed condition and to progress the body towards inner balance and healthy vitality.

Generally, the healing crisis is a much misunderstood activity – or range of activities – performed by your body when it seeks to maintain or to regain good health. The term 'crisis' is perhaps unfortunate as it tends to be synonymous with catastrophe; in this case it means nothing more than a turning point. There are other therapies that recognise the concept of the healing crisis but few, if any, of them see it as such a vital part of the body's overall *maintenance* of health.

It can be difficult to comprehend that fevers, cold, sickness, and diarrhoea could ever be beneficial. How can these unpleasant episodes be seen as cleansing efforts? The last two more obviously can as the body ejects unwanted food from the alimentary tract but the first two can be explained as a 'bonfire' effect. A combustion or clearing away of accumulated rubbish that is hindering normal bodily activity. We believe that two common colds a year are as effective a guarantee as one can get against more serious illness

– with the important proviso that you allow the waste to exit successfully and don't attempt to suppress the clear out.

Cardiff University Common Cold Research[1] Department found that:

> Despite the fact that very few of us escape from at least a couple of common cold infections each year, common cold viruses are not very contagious. Under laboratory conditions when healthy volunteers are kept with others who are suffering from common cold infections it has proven remarkably difficult to spread infection from one person to another.

We often hear people talk of catching a cold but with our years of clinical experience and the above finding we can, with some confidence, say that colds are usually simple forms of healing crises and as such have a beneficial effect on your body if allowed to follow their full and natural course. The Common Cold research department doesn't offer any cures – just a list of symptom suppressants. As we have already identified, the action of suppressing symptoms is not helpful to the organism, your body, as a whole, even if it might give you temporary relief from a runny nose or a stuffed up head.

The crisis, or turning point, is fundamental to your progress from ill health to vigorous rude health, particularly as it is possible that some symptoms can be exacerbated on the principle of 'getting worse before getting better' after a period of treatment. The Healing Crisis is a real test of confidence. My uncle says, 'coax the patient to jump this fence and the race is theirs'.

Some people are incredulous when it is pointed out that the

---

1   The Cardiff University Common Cold Centre. www.cardiff.ac.uk

LIVE WELL. EAT WELL. BE WELL.

body prefers to be healthy and in balance and will, through the activity of our vital organs, do its level best to maintain optimum functionality despite our apparent worst efforts to thwart it. If everything is equal – which let's face it, it rarely is – and if we come from a healthy family with a good genetic make-up, and if our nutrition is well balanced and wholesome, and if the air we breathe is clean, and if the water we drink is pure, and if our work is fulfilling and pays us enough to have a decent roof over our heads, and if our family relationships are harmonious, and if we are creative, and fit from regular exercise – preferably in the fresh air – then homeostasis (a state of internal equilibrium) can be maintained for some time without need for a healing crisis. But, let's face it, how many of us are fortunate enough to enjoy a life with all those advantages? Not many of us can achieve all of the above during our lifetimes, never mind concurrently. The best we can do is to eat sensibly, to remember to breathe deeply, to walk when we can, make enough money to keep the bills at bay whilst, if we're really lucky, doing something we love.

Looked at another way: the civilised human's troubles generally arise from their failure to meet their body's simple basic requirements. When an individual tries to cheat the system on a regular basis the body will eventually protest, and then when things go wrong the body is blamed for letting them down. Not content with that unfairness, the individual will go on to punish their body with poison and even mutilation under the euphemism of 'treatment'; and all this in the attempt to find a cure.

Our bodies are incredibly adaptable and tolerant of our little bad habits, they permit us a huge amount of latitude, a fact that most of us take full advantage of. We push the boundaries when we can but somehow we still maintain a reasonable level of health. So where does the healing crisis come in? There can be any number of reasons why the body decides that it must do something about the toxic build-up in our tissues, the tipping point is as unique as the individual, and often the 'bug doing the rounds' is enough to instigate the required activity.

Our cleansing organs, the liver, kidneys, lungs and skin deal continually with the waste products produced by our bodies. If you are working within your energy limits and free from stress then the body can keep on top of this work, but if you are doing too much, or not getting enough sleep or under stress then the system can be compromised and a little waste gets stored to be dealt with later. Put simply, when there is a backlog, the body has to make an extra effort to deal with it.

Cleansing activities

Genuine wholesomeness and efficiency in your body systems are not sustained without vital effort, and the cleanliness of every single cell of the living body is one of the major tasks for our vital life forces. It is often likened to the never ending job of housework in keeping the home clean, and some prefer to call the healing crisis 'the body's spring-clean'. But whatever you choose to call it, why should such repeated – and occasionally almost violent – cleaning activity be necessary, particularly if you are living a healthy life? To begin with, even the most wholesome foods you eat and the cleanest air you breathe brings some impurity into your body. For most of us, foods are far from wholesome and the atmosphere is more or less contaminated, so that these two factors alone might be enough to necessitate an occasional extraordinary bodily cleansing effort. But in so many cases the existing burdens are added to by any number of extra stresses, these days they can range from excessive work commitments, to money worries and relationship problems. Our excretory and blood-cleansing organs deal with the wastes that result from daily metabolic and digestive processes, and these wastes are usually dealt with easily. In equitable conditions, this work is well within the capabilities of the organs. So great are the natural reserves that it is usual for only a moderate proportion of the working cells to be in action at any given time: the remainder are effectively resting and recuperating. However, if these organs are compromised or overworked, wastes start to build up in the tissues

Internal equilibrium can exist only so long as there is no external hindrance, so long as the individual's way of living has some semblance of balance, and so long as the cleansing organs are assured a sufficient supply of good quality essential materials. Given these in suitable amounts, the tissues that form the flesh, the bones and the vital organs of the body have almost unbelievable potential for self-repair and maintenance. They have ample resources to meet day-to-day wear and tear, and most forms of accidental injury.

Dr John Henry Tilden in his book 'Toxaemia Explained'[2] recognised that:

> Dis-ease of the organism occurs when the waste products
> of normal cell metabolism cannot be expelled as quickly as
> they are being produced, and accumulations of potentially
> toxic waste are instead stored in the adjacent tissues.

This toxic state of the tissues is exactly the pre-existing condition that the virus or 'bad' bacteria is looking for, just the 'soil' that 'the bug that is doing the rounds' is seeking to accommodate its

---

2   Tilden, Dr John Henry (1851–1940) Toxaemia Explained.
     www.soilandhealth.org

proliferation. There does not necessarily need to be any obvious external stimuli, your somatic intelligence may have simply made the decision for itself, it may have recognised that the situation was no longer tenable. So your healthy body could be reacting to those 'invading' organisms or it could simply be reacting to the unacceptable build-up of excess toxic wastes and a Healing Crisis will ensue. The Healing Crisis can take many forms; most of them are unpleasant, and the timing is rarely convenient. How often have you gotten ill when you have taken some leave from work? Ruing the fact that you are in bed feeling awful when you had all sorts of interesting activities scheduled.

My grandfather, James C Thomson, wrote of the Healing Crisis and its role in health:

> Real health is rarely placid. As a rule it is a study in dynamics and every now and again it can assume an aspect of sheer violence. This exuberance makes for misunderstanding. People mistake healthy reactions for disease and try to stop them; particularly as health phenomena are not generally studied. Indeed, except by the Nature Cure School, health, as such, is not investigated. The usual acceptance is that health is a negative quality – a mere absence of symptoms of disease. This conception is ludicrously false.
>
> Consider a man who has swallowed a deadly fungus. If he is in a state of virile health his reaction will be sickness and diarrhoea. Not merely nausea, but a vigorous and complete emptying of the stomach and bowels. The better the health of the individual involved, the more decisive will be this demonstration of house-cleaning.
>
> The first point to notice is that the more thorough and immediate the evacuation, the less will be the damage done

to the patient. Anything which would soothe and nullify the expulsive effort would be deadly to the man, no matter how kindly and scientifically applied. It is a point of no little importance that the more efficient the method used, the more dangerous it would be for the patient.

The poisoning of an individual from the ingestion of a noxious substance is a very obvious instance, but it is an illustration of the Nature Cure reasoning as applied to acute conditions. Exactly the same philosophy applies in more complicated circumstances. For instance, rather than the poison being ingested, it has instead gathered slowly in any organ where it cannot be expelled by normal excretory activity or simple sickness. This is the toxaemia that Dr Tilden talked of, and a point is reached where the local tissues start a more radical cleaning-out, and this activity can take any one of a number of forms. The simple cold or diarrhoea, the more specialised rash or abscess, or an effort involving the whole of the body's forces, such as a fever; one and all have the same purpose. All are indications of the body's healing and cleansing efforts and its striving towards a state of good health.

Stored wastes and their toxic effects

So, will you know when you are in a toxic state? That is a difficult question; the signs or symptoms will be as unique as the individual who is experiencing them. The body is ingenious in its ability to store wastes in little-used areas of non-vital structures. Often the accumulations are so gradual and your energy levels diminish so slowly that these wastes might lie unnoticed for years or become more and more apparent as in the slow onset of rheumatoid arthritis. As the effects are cumulative and insidious, our lack of vitality is reduced so gradually that it can take some time before the full extent of the burden is realised.

Sometimes the toxic overload is diffused almost uniformly, so that you might be aware of getting a bit overweight but otherwise have no real symptoms; but this form of oedema is a signpost to strain within your system. The blood stream itself may be carrying a constant burden of excess toxic wastes, which it is lugging around in the vain hope that one or other of the eliminative organs may be able to accept and dispose of it.

If your blood is overloaded in this way, it is less able to carry the freshly oxygenated air from your lungs to all of your body tissues; also it is less able to take in the waste products from those tissues and its ability to transport nutrients is compromised. It is thickened and sluggish, so that your heart is forced to work harder than normal. The heart muscle itself relies upon that same blood for nourishment and cleansing and so do the blood carrying vessels. So you can see that it is only a matter of time before these structures too, must show signs of fatigue and ultimately disorder or breakdown.

Throughout this gradual drift away from normality, there will have been repeated warnings which you will probably have largely disregarded or medicated into submission, and they will be in the form of colds, flu, general discomforts, headaches, stiffness, pains and disturbed organ function. But, being either ignored or knocked out with pain killing and sedative drugs, the sentinel nerve centres may become discouraged and their sensitivity lost. When this happens you can easily become dejected and apathetic. Alternatively, the concentrations of toxic wastes around the nerves may rise so that these make known their anguish only too clearly. Your joints may lose their mobility, bones may even become mis-shapen, muscles lose their strength and elasticity, tumours make their presence known. Clarity of thought, too, is often a victim of toxic overload, and you might find yourself progressively less able to cope with people and situations. Some of these signs may provoke you to take action: but too often this can take the form of seeking a comforting palliative drug.

It can be difficult to see how such seemingly trivial things as everyday bad habits and an accumulation of toxic wastes can lead logically to total and premature breakdown, particularly if you are viewing the situation from an orthodox angle. But this is where cause and effect are at work, and the earlier the causes of your distress are addressed then the sooner you can stop the progression from healthy normality. The more basic vitality that you still have, the brighter the prospects of a reasonable recovery. But is it really possible for the body to lift itself out of a truly unpleasant state of toxicity, internal chaos and emotional depression?

Encouragement and Reassurance

Rest assured, we are not expecting you to be able to cope with your illness on your own, self-reliant though Nature Cure people tend to be, and we are certainly not expecting you to deal with your first Healing Crisis without support and advice. If you are in a really poor state then you must consult a Nature Cure practitioner. Your practitioner may employ any number of methods – massage and manipulation, water treatment, fasting, psychology, food reform, exercise, controlled sunbathing – the aim is to help you understand how you have arrived at this situation and to move your body to take effective action. If you are on medication then there will be dialogue between you and, if necessary, your doctor to reduce and, preferably, eventually stop that medication. Apart from that, just what form the actions might take depends upon many things, not least of which are your reserves of vital energy and your personality. What matters here is the ultimate effect of treatment; helping your body to start a vigorous and effective effort to rid itself of the accumulated debris. When this happens, the exciting and encouraging result is the Healing Crisis.

Of course us Nature Cure practitioners don't claim any exclusive rights to instigating the Healing Crisis: as mentioned above it can be initiated without any obvious external stimulus. So how does that happen? Well, if you have made some positive changes in your way of living then there might just be enough of a rise in the level of your vitality available for the necessary repair work to start. It can also occur – and it often does – in the form of some acute illness that is 'doing the rounds'. As explained earlier, for a circulating contagious illness to take hold your tissues have to be in the right condition for the virus or bacteria to proliferate. It should not be disregarded that what many of us perceive as an ordinary cold is in fact a simple and potentially effective form of healing crisis. I say 'potentially' because it is so important that the cleansing effort is not suppressed if the somatic activities are to have a positive outcome. However, we are for the moment more concerned with the less usual type of eliminative effort – remarkable for its vigour or its nature – which occurs as a result of deliberate encouragement.

The actual healing crisis

So how will you know if you are having a healing crisis? Don't doubt it for a minute – you will know! It might feel like the world is ending but trust your body to know what it is doing, after all, it was ignoring its endless warnings that got you to this point, now it's time for some humility and to give some credit to that amazing innate intelligence. You need to give your body all the help you can, but how do you do that?

There are two main ways in which your body may adapt itself to deal with tasks too great for the normal cleansing organs to cope with. In the first way your body sacrifices, temporarily, your normal functions. These are often the delicate and complex activities that we know as conscious intelligence and reasoning. This happens as your system departs from the usually closely regulated conditions that make them possible. Your body temperature is allowed to rise a few degrees and this enables many vital processes to be considerably sped-up. You will feel fevered and, consequently, unable to perform your normal mental and physical work. But, just as an insect or reptile is more lively in warm weather than in cold, so the cells of the body can carry out a great deal of work in a comparatively short time. My grandmother described the fever as a bonfire for the body. *Bon fire* – good fire.

In addition, in your fevered condition you will have little or no interest in food and you will want to be left quietly alone. This is no small matter, since it means that your energy is conserved for the immediate and vital processes of the Healing Crisis. The energy, which you would have otherwise expended on digestion, is instead available for collecting, conveying, processing, filtering and eliminating all the excess wastes. And, as it has been estimated that digestion absorbs more energy than any other everyday activity in the average person, this saving alone is significant.

Ordinarily, a feverish crisis of this type does not extend beyond two or three days and is often much shorter. Yet during this brief time, your body may catch up with many months' accumulation of wastes. In this form of crisis, nothing extraordinary occurs, other than the aforementioned suspension of intellectual ability. In addition to this, little or no physical effort will be required beyond taking the odd sip of water and getting as much sleep and rest as possible. This allows the normal blood cleansing organs to carry out the eliminative work, in their normal way, but working a little harder than usual.

Uncomfortable symptoms

There are other ways that the Healing Crisis can manifest and these conditions can have many and varied superficial appearances, but an essential feature is the adaptation of some bodily tissue or organ for waste-elimination. The kinds of crisis activity are not at all exclusive; they may occur side by side or in sequence, but it may make the situation easier to understand if their respective characteristics are recognised.

A common presentation of a Healing Crisis may be seen and felt as swelling of your glands. In this instance one or more of the activities of glandular structures are temporarily diverted from their normal functions to become emergency 'decontaminators' and there is generally a rise in your temperature.

Another variety is most easily observed in such forms as skin eruptions and rashes, through which the accumulations of rubbish are ejected directly from the body into the outside world, or in catarrh, where the mucus membranes eliminate wastes in the way of discoloured phlegm. Your skin reorganises its functions to permit a more massive outflow than occurs in normal perspiration and sebaceous secretion. With a catarrhal crisis the linings of your nose, throat and upper breathing tubes excrete wastes as well as the normal cleansing and protective flow of mucus.

The intensity of effort may vary all the way from a mild rash to a crop of pustules; from a cold in the head to a choking sore throat. Yet, no matter how violent the symptoms, how raging the fever or how seemingly destructive the effects, if you can accept their importance in the cleaning process then you will see these upheavals as the body's drastic efforts to rid itself of accumulated wastes and toxins which are threatening your vital and normal function.

Calculation

The intensity of your body's activity is an indicator of just how desperate a condition your body must have been. However, at all times, the total intelligence of the system is in control. It is continually weighing up conflicting demands and making decisions that favour long-term, vital survival. In severe cases it may even sacrifice the most easily repaired or least essential tissues in order to conserve and protect the irreplaceable and truly vital. In the most extreme cases, a proportion of the active tissue of a vital organ may have to be sacrificed, and it can be very hard for the orthodoxly trained onlooker to stand by and do nothing. Yet one must do just that, allowing the individual body to compute its own schedule on the basis of innumerable factors of which no human being can be consciously aware, far less be able to correlate. This all sounds very frightening, but the alternative it to suppress the symptoms, deluge your body with toxic substances, suffer a range of side-effects and actually end up apparently recovering and feeling better, until your next breakdown.

Interference

The well-meaning bystander, and this can be a spouse; a family member or good friend, is potentially the greatest stumbling block in the whole situation. Their fear of the situation, which is generally based on an orthodox understanding, causes anxiety that makes them feel rather helpless and that 'something must be done'. This is an entirely understandable situation but you must hold fast and do all you can to reassure them that everything is under control.

Whether the well-meant gesture is encouragement to eat or a more sophisticated disruption of the body's plans and actions with drugs and antibiotics, any 'helpful' interference could end up obstructing your body's true healing potential.

Effort

It may not be easy to discontinue all the little unhelpful daily habits that have contributed to your condition of disease. In themselves, each one is probably not that bad really, but added together they build up to quite a burden. Errors in diet, clothing that is restricting or prevents the skin from functioning at its best, your posture – sitting hunched over a computer for hours on end in a stuffy office – prescription and non-prescription drugs and a few destructive mental attitudes thrown in for good measure, are all common factors. Hopefully you will have become so fed up feeling unwell that prospects of starting new and interesting ways of living will provide enough encouragement to take the first steps. Some simple changes to your daily habits and routines should see a reduction in the intake of stimulants, processed foods and alcohol, coupled with an increase in exercise, deep breathing and more walking in the fresh air. Consequently there will be fewer residues of wastes needing to be transported and handled and this means that your bloodstream and its associated cleansing organs are able to function more efficiently and within healthy parameters. General exercise, such as walking, as well as specific exercises, can help to undo existing damage and rebuild healthy tissues. But care

LIVE WELL. EAT WELL. BE WELL.

must be taken not to overdo the trips to the gym, and to avoid over fussiness with your new diet; over enthusiasm in the early days can quickly wane and interest is lost. Nature Cure isn't a quick fix solution to get better so that you can resume your previous damaging habits; it is a fundamental life change that will mean that the bad habits are not so enticing any more and good health will be the 'fix'. In some cases manipulative treatment may be needed to make a more complete job of correcting postural weaknesses. And last, but by no means least, a better understanding of your emotional conflicts can so often resolve tensions that notoriously waste nervous energy at an alarming rate.

Intolerance of not feeling well

One thing that you will notice, and might resent at first, is that the more positive changes you make to your daily habits the more sensitive your body will become to unacceptable internal conditions. Where before a heavy weekend of overeating, not enough sleep and too much alcohol might have just resulted in a Monday morning muzzy head, your new found cleaner and clearer system will protest more loudly and you will quickly learn to adjust to its protestations. Any accumulations of wastes will not be tolerated by your newly appreciated somatic sense and your conscious self will quickly be made aware of those wastes accumulations too. Gradually, both you and your tissues begin to regain self-respect and, with it, there is an increasing intolerance of any substandard state of the body. The reduction in stored waste and toxins gives the system a chance, effectively, to get back its breath and to take stock. The improved – less obstructed – circulation of blood and oxygen and flow of nervous energy have re-invigorated the vital organs. The more generous supply of nutrients and of potentially acid-absorbing materials swings the chemical balances in the direction of greater vital activity. (See the chapter 'What To Eat For Health' for dietary suggestions.) The deepening conviction that something constructive is happening and a better appreciation of values allows you to develop greater ambition, confidence and contentment.

All these fundamental changes work together, consciously and unconsciously, to ensure a positive outcome from a well handled Healing Crisis. Gradually, your body will work out its plan of action and set out on the series of activities that will allow it to achieve its true potential. Each organ will have its part to play, and every tissue will have extra work to perform – it might be only an increase of normal function or it could be the taking on of some special, emergency task. The somatic intelligence must be allowed to decide upon a scale of priorities: it cannot hope to eliminate 20 years' accumulation of ingrained waste in a few days, and it must give first consideration to the most vital tissues. For instance the first Healing Crisis often seems to produce no improvement at all in the symptom that most annoys you – for example a stiff or painful joint – yet it clears away some strain or obstruction from a truly vital organ. As a rough guide (this can vary greatly with individuals) about six weeks elapse between the initiation of reformed living habits and the first sign of crisis activity. A few youngsters, with basically good vitality, may produce a first-class healing crisis within five weeks.

Crisis features a few words of caution

The Healing Crisis may also be recognised by various character-istics. The six-week interval is an indication in some cases, but probably the most consistent feature, as recognised during 50

LIVE WELL. EAT WELL. BE WELL.

years of clinical experience in the Kingston Clinic, is the individual's statement that 'this is exactly the trouble I had years ago!' It has often been expressed in those very words, with understandable overtones of incredulity and doubt. The individual is quite right; the body is now returning to tasks which were previously interrupted or frustrated by suppressive treatment, or by lack of available vital energy. The healing crisis is your body's opportunity to carry the jobs at least one step nearer to achieving rude health.

Another common phenomenon is a wonderful experience of exhilaration for a day or two before the healing crisis starts. This feeling is often misleadingly intense, and even for those who have had a few healing crises, it is at first welcomed as the opportunity to conquer the world before the truth dawns. However, it does indicate that your body is confidently preparing for the big event. We have to remember – and this is the difficult bit – not to waste the energy that is so obviously plentiful on non-vital exertions. It is not always easy to persuade someone, who has perhaps for years been handicapped in some way, to forgo the pleasure of exercising his or her newfound vigour. Carried away by enthusiasm and the enjoyment of a level of energy not felt for years they will, for example, go off and climb a high hill after being previously limited to gentle, level walks. Admirable as this may seem at the time, sadly it can mean burning up energy that was intended for healing and repair. If this sounds like a very pessimistic view, it isn't. Once you understand the Healing Crisis and how it works you will accept the buzz the days before, go through the unpleasant symptoms during the cleaning out period and reap the benefit of a cleaner system afterwards. Nothing is instant, but hang on in there and enjoy the clearer head and happier body later.

The duration and intensity of any healing crisis is extremely variable. As a general rule, the more vital the individual, the shorter and more vigorous the episode will be. The person with reduced vitality may have to be content with a more restrained, and possibly prolonged, crisis. Every bodily house cleaning is a strictly individual experience and, apart from some recurrence of old symptoms, it is not possible to forecast accurately the sequence of events in a crisis. An experienced Nature Cure practitioner may have a pretty fair inkling of probabilities, but to predict is risky for two reasons: if they estimate falsely, the patient's confidence may be lost; if correctly, there may have been an influence on the course of the crisis by suggestion. The latter could so easily be seen as an unfortunate interference.

To completion

The anticipation of another Healing Crisis seems to worry patients in their first few months of Nature Cure living. It is very likely that things got unexpectedly intense during their first Healing Crisis, and there may be a sneaking feeling that they were lucky to escape unscathed from it. Yet the essential fact – to be grasped and firmly held – is that your body is in confident control of the whole situation, knowing exactly what its reserves are and how much it can attempt without risk of lasting damage. The body wants to be healthy, it will do all it can to move towards that state, and it might do some apparently strange and difficult-to-understand things to achieve that goal.

A calm, understanding acceptance that the whole process must be allowed to run its full course without interruption is essential. Here is a simple analogy that my father liked to use (although like all analogies it has limited application). Take a roller coaster ride at a theme park. For most of us, a journey on it has moments of terror and distress; yet through it all we have the assurance that it was engineered by competent builders, that the dangers are more apparent than real, and that if we just sit tight we shall arrive safely and happily at the planned destination. That a switchback ride brings us back to our starting point and achieves nothing constructive bears little resemblance to a true Healing Crisis, but in other ways, it has striking similarities. First, there is the slow, laborious and uneventful climb to the necessary height, that breathless moment just before the plunge, then a succession of drops, bumps, jolts and threatened terrors. Probably most significant of all, there is the vitally important proviso: 'Everything will be alright if we just sit tight.'

No matter how alarmed you might feel, it would make no sense to attempt to get off the rollercoaster during one of its sickening plunges. It is perfectly obvious that this would be dangerous in the extreme. Yet, when confronted by a comparable situation within your own body, it is sorely tempting to choose to make a quick exit. Sadly, it is likely that you will be encouraged to do so by over-concerned friends and relations. These well-meaning folk see it as their duty to warn you of your peril, and caution of all the terrible events that may befall you unless you change your course. However, if you were to try to step out then, whether by accepting unwanted food or by having some vital activity interrupted with drugs, the results will be the opposite of a properly conducted Healing Crisis. If you do decide to abandon your resolve and take your friend's advice your decision may not be immediately life threatening, but there will be a cost. There will be a further weakening of your constitution and the accumulated wastes will still be hampering your system. Your vital organs that were tuned and committed to healing and cleaning activity are left less able to protect themselves against massive interference from outside. Even a relatively 'simple' drug – such as an aspirin or a laxative – may produce apparent instant relief but the actual outcome is damaging, more so if you have started to become less accustomed to taking medication.

How long will it all take?

As a very rough guide, one month of careful attention to your diet, exercise and lifestyle per year of unhelpful and disease producing habits is usually enough to allow the body to re-regulate itself and find a better balance.

Bodily spring-cleanings may take place comparatively frequently – approximately at six-week intervals – and with varying intensity until the whole system has reached a reasonable and workable state of wholesomeness. The form of the crisis may suggest a 'illness with a name' or it may be more simply a succession of obviously eliminative activities.

Above all, the bodily spring-clean is not a thing to fear any more than its domestic equivalent. It should ideally be earnestly worked for, and once brought into action it should be welcomed and allowed to run its full, unimpeded course. It is literally a rejuvenating process and an encouraging experience. As your body becomes healthier you will start to experience the true effects of a Healing Crisis well handled. Better clarity of thought, more energy, more vitality and a better emotional balance.

So what should you do when experiencing a Healing Crisis? Basically, think what any wild animal would do. Snuggle down in a warm, safe place, have a window open to keep the air fresh, don't eat anything and have only sips of plain water. The body needs all the energy it can get to proceed with its vital work. If you are fevered or headachy or your glands are swollen then some relief can be gained from the use of cold-water compresses round your neck and waist without impeding somatic activity. In fact, the waist compress can be very helpful during a Healing Crisis and offers some relaxation and often better sleep. See the chapter on Water and Nature Cure for full explanations of how to make and use compresses and what they do and how they work. If you are unsure about any aspect of this please consult a qualified Nature Cure practitioner.

So is there a downside?

A downside? Well, as a lifelong Nature Cure person I can put my hand on my heart and say – 'Yes'. It is the guilt trip! It is completely non-productive but still it happens. The 'if only' self-berating starts to occupy the mind. If only I hadn't done this or that, or over eaten this or that or overdone whatever. Ditch the negative thoughts, what is done is done, the body is dealing with it and just remember to take more care in future. As mentioned before, the body will protest much more quickly and vigorously to an unacceptable situation when it is truly vital and healthy.

Points to remember

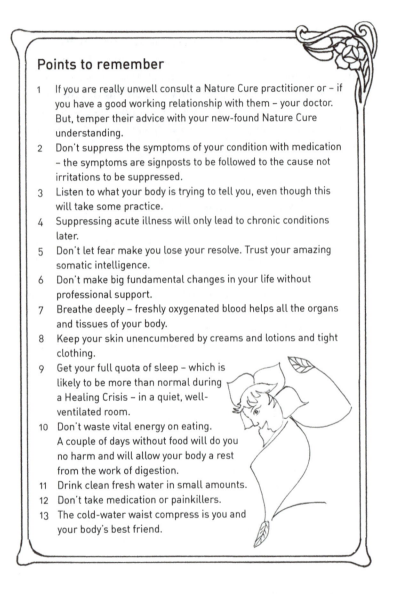

1　If you are really unwell consult a Nature Cure practitioner or – if you have a good working relationship with them – your doctor. But, temper their advice with your new-found Nature Cure understanding.

2　Don't suppress the symptoms of your condition with medication – the symptoms are signposts to be followed to the cause not irritations to be suppressed.

3　Listen to what your body is trying to tell you, even though this will take some practice.

4　Suppressing acute illness will only lead to chronic conditions later.

5　Don't let fear make you lose your resolve. Trust your amazing somatic intelligence.

6　Don't make big fundamental changes in your life without professional support.

7　Breathe deeply – freshly oxygenated blood helps all the organs and tissues of your body.

8　Keep your skin unencumbered by creams and lotions and tight clothing.

9　Get your full quota of sleep – which is likely to be more than normal during a Healing Crisis – in a quiet, well-ventilated room.

10　Don't waste vital energy on eating. A couple of days without food will do you no harm and will allow your body a rest from the work of digestion.

11　Drink clean fresh water in small amounts.

12　Don't take medication or painkillers.

13　The cold-water waist compress is you and your body's best friend.

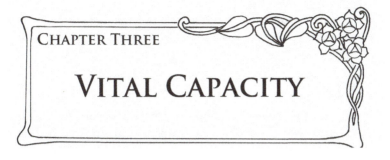

CHAPTER THREE

VITAL CAPACITY

MY FATHER WAS often asked how a person who has lived a Nature Cure life for 50 years can develop a degenerative disease. It seems a simple question, yet its implications are challenging, and there is no straight answer. If you look at the individual's life in its totality it is usually possible to find lots of reasons. The question carries a potentially misleading implication. It suggests that Nature Cure can promise you, or anyone, a total freedom from serious disorder and a life far longer than that of 'ordinary' people. This is to misunderstand the human condition.

All life depends upon vitality and it can be described variously as exuberant physical strength, mental vigour, a good capacity for survival or the power to live and grow. But vitality is not elastic, it is not a purchasable commodity and you cannot buy more of it if you run out. It is a substance or 'stuff' that each one of us inherits in a finite quantity when we are born, and we consume it as we live our lives. Our individual inheritance of vitality depends largely upon our parents, they provide our genetic inheritance, but the rate at which we consume it depends greatly on our own temperament and our chosen lifestyle. So it follows that a good start in life, coupled with a sensible way of living, with a few doses of good luck and providence along the way, offers the best prospect for a long, useful and rewarding life. Poor heredity and abnormal pressures or stresses, accidental injury or other factors can result in a markedly reduced capacity for individual fulfilment or achievement.

The young

Ideally our job should be to advise prospective parents how to ensure that their chosen lifestyle will give their children the best chance of healthy productive lives. When the next generation is born our undertaking should also include teaching that new life how to make the best use of its vital resources. Sadly, it is much more often the case that our task is to attempt to rescue the older individual from the confusions that their life has thrown up. Our efforts then go into addressing their maladies and how they can make the best use of their remaining, often sadly depleted, vitality.

At this stage it should be clarified that *vitality* is not the same thing as *energy*. The two are interrelated, it is true, but do not necessarily correspond. So far as they can be interlinked, it could be said that good vitality is the ability to produce plenty of energy throughout a long lifetime. But reduced vitality does not necessarily limit energy output over a brief interval. Indeed, it can often lead to an excessive production of energy used up in relatively short bursts. An illustration of this would be the musicians and artists who have produced their most intensively compelling work while in desperate physical decline. This naturally raises the question: was it worth it? But only the individual concerned has the right to answer that, and their answer is valid whether the rest of the world considers them to be insane or a genius.

Punishment

As we have already explained, individual vitality cannot be restored once it has been consumed, but in practice excellent and workable recoveries from desperate illness can be achieved. Learning to compensate and conserve your resources can be extraordinarily difficult; we can all be blind to our own stubbornness and resistance to change, even when we easily see these attitudes in others.

The relationship, and lack thereof, between energy and vitality can be illustrated by showing the difference between quality and power. We have all bought items that are well made, work within the limits of their capacity, and last for years and years. We will also have bought cheap items that are not so well made but blast away to their limits before self-destructing – usually at an inconvenient time. In a similar way, if the structural quality – the vitality – of an individual is well matched to their energy, then they will be a balanced person. Just as there are, for instance, small cars of modest power that go on and on – because their limited structural strength is not overstrained – so there are people who have not even an average vitality, yet who quietly live long and useful lives. Others can put up incredibly energetic performances – giving the impression of superhuman power – but they have a way of suddenly collapsing at what should be middle age.

The similarities go further because, as well as tissue quality and power-producing capacity, there is the all-important factor of the controlling intelligence. To use the car analogy again, a good steady driver can make a modest vehicle last and with some regular maintenance that vehicle can deliver a creditable performance. By comparison a hashy or impatient driver will destroy even the finest machinery in a remarkably short time. So if you can recognise your physical limitations, accept the need for proper fuel (food and fresh air) and maintenance (sleep and rest), plus a reasonable regard for the rules of cause and effect, you will go a long way towards achieving a healthy and productive life.

Toxic effects

Vitality is consumed in many ways, often insidiously. Often this is caused by the common belief that there is a lower limit below which such things as tea, coffee, tobacco, alcohol and other popular drugs do us no harm. Broadly this may appear to be true, because there are no outward signs to the contrary, no ailment occurs which is obviously connected with the habit and the individual lives a long life without any obviously attributable ill health. The operative word here is 'obviously', because all stimulant or toxic substances taken into your body must consume vitality, even if in too small a quantity to be noticed immediately. The only convincing test for most people is direct comparison or a double blind trial, and this is almost impossible to apply. Individuals vary so much in their constitutions that it may be pointless to compare the levels of function between one subject taking four cups of coffee a day with that of another not taking any. Further to this, other factors may completely swamp any observable effects which a toxic substance or destructive habit produces. The only true comparison, and this too has its limitations, is to record the behaviour and wellbeing of the same individual over two longish intervals – say, five or ten years each – during which the two contrasting ways of living are adhered to. Despite the slowness and uncertainty of such a method, significant patterns do emerge as the decades pass. 'Decades! Who cares about ten-year intervals these days, when everything must be instant?' My father wrote that plaintive sentence in 1969 long before our fast-moving, and genuinely almost instant, world of emails and texts.

Experienced practitioners of Nature Cure can often estimate vitality in individuals. But while the appearance and behaviour of a newcomer to Nature Cure speaks volumes, we have to be aware of those who have learned how to put on a good show. An apparent high output of energy will impress us, as will their clear enthusiasm, but we have to try to see beyond these. If the physique does not quite seem to match the performance we are right to be suspicious. Although to be a vital person you don't necessarily need to be of robust build, if there is not sufficient room in the body cavity for vital organs of ample size there must be some limitation. Some people of slender build tend to lack vitality, but there are also the 'wiry' types whose lack of bulk is misleading. Usually, these are individuals who learned early in life that barely enough is far better than a feast, and who have thus avoided vital overload. Their seemingly limited capacity is ample for their needs, and they can call on good vital reserves to meet emergencies when necessary. This is as good an excuse as any to offer some wise words on the benefits of moderation (by an unknown author): 'You can eat just so much in a life time, and the sooner you eat it the sooner you die'.

Build

Individuals of sturdy build usually have an adequate set of vital organs and the development of the chest usually reflects the capacity of the lungs, as well as the potential of the heart. Well-supported abdominal contents – preferably without fatty deposits – suggest ample digestive and metabolic capabilities. The emotional responses of the individual can also offer us useful clues; Irritability, or a tendency to be offended by innocent remarks, betrays insecurity and this may be due to insufficient vital reserves. On the other hand, unusual tolerance might be an indication of a further stage of decline – the individual is 'past caring'. Often, the Nature Cure practitioner will have to delay their interpretations until they know their patient better. As time goes on the patient's guard will come down, at which point their true condition can be properly assessed and worked with honestly.

The development of the arms and legs and the general muscular build are unreliable as indications of vital capacity. This is mainly because these can be affected by the usual activities of the individual, both professional and recreational, as well as by inherent vitality. A sprinter or weight lifter may have enormous muscles, but have only a moderate vital capacity. The long-distance athlete, however, usually has comparatively slender limbs coupled with well-developed vital organs.

Even if you have a good grasp of the principles of Nature Cure, and attempt to apply them to your everyday life, you are not afforded any secret store of vitality. We all have to accept the limits of our own vital capacities. Any person with poor heredity, or a history of serious childhood or early-life illness – particularly illnesses which may have caused damage to vital tissues or organs – cannot expect to live as full a life as a comparable individual who had an altogether better start. Many people find it hard to believe or accept that the past cannot be completely wiped out, but it can be seen as a tremendous tribute to Nature Cure's success that those with reduced vitality are given the ability to live productive and active lives.

Ourselves

We are all prone to forgetfulness and, often misplaced, optimism, particularly if the realities are uncomfortable to face. So when a group of Nature Cure practitioners gather together, and we look around, we are liable to ask ourselves 'what is so special about being us?' We are not outstandingly free from illness and we all show signs of ageing. Some of our numbers even die without having reached a remarkable age. If this is the best we can do, what should we expect from our patients? Answer: at least as much as we have, on average, achieved for ourselves, and in many cases we may justifiably expect a great deal more.

Many individual practitioners came to Nature Cure in the first place because they were desperately ill. The history of Nature Cure is littered with those who first experienced it as a way to save their own lives – if not from an immediate threat of extinction, then from a progressive deterioration. That these threats no longer cause fear does not alter the essential facts: the case history may be forgotten, but the damage previously done to vital organs and the early excessive consumption of vitality have left a permanent deficiency.

Taking things for granted

Our unconscious somatic intelligence is repeatedly shocked by the idiotic things our 'educated' mentality does. We behave in ways that show a total disregard for the warnings that our deep, vital intelligence is constantly trying to give us. If we take our health and an expected resilience for granted, our conscious selves are often working against our somatic intelligence. The more we 'behave ourselves' according to the inescapable rules of our physical existence, the more fully and effectively our bodies will co-operate with our conscious selves and the better our health will be.

So what affects the vital capacity of an individual? Age is important, and some allowances will need to be made as the individual ages. Younger children always seem to have plenty of vitality and this often enables them to bounce back to full vigour after a setback, however lengthy. It is the late teenagers and young adults who are most likely to be concerned by any evidence of physical limitations. They worry when their constitution does not seem to be able keep up with their chosen lifestyle, but it is often possible to help and support them to make the small changes to their lives that enables them to adapt to and enjoy a fulfilling life.

Stability

Once early adulthood is passed, if the individual adopts a reasonably sensible way of life, for most people there appears to be a plateau of fairly consistent health, which can last some 30 to 40 years. For instance, rapid dental deterioration in the teens may give way to comparative stability of the remaining teeth, as hearty appetites sated with junk food and caffeine drinks grow into more sensible and balanced diets.

So much depends on each individual's attitude to lifestyle choices, and the picture can be totally skewed by medication, surgery or other unnatural treatments. It is quite possible that damage can be caused and situations created early on that make consistent good health in later life more difficult. Nature Cure always aims to make the fullest possible use of any available vitality but there will be times when that quantity seems rather limited. For an individual who has become dependent on drugs that burn up vitality in order to produce an appearance of improvement, the realities can be harsh. No one who has undergone, or closely observed, the effects of steroids such as cortisone should need any further convincing of that.

It is usually at some time after middle age that most of us start to become aware of our vital limitations. There is a growing realisation that we can no longer force ourselves to carry through exceptional tasks, when formerly we would have cheerfully roared into action. The initial flow of energy soon dwindles, in some exceptionally determined individuals the self-imposed task is performed in their usual energetic way, and then they are horrified to find themselves lacking in energy for several days afterwards.

Stimulants

The solution turned to, too often, is an increasing dependence upon stimulants. A constant driving of the body beyond natural capabilities and supplies means that some way has to be found of making remaining vital reserves more readily available. This is when what are commonly accepted as relatively harmless stimulants begin to become insidious. A cup of tea or coffee drunk socially probably causes the system a minimum of distress and might even be beneficial, but it is when the hard-driven individual begins to feel they must soon have another cup that the addiction starts to become established. More and more cups are swallowed, to increasingly disruptive effect; caffeine is rated as the most popular psychoactive drug in the world. The active ingredients in tea and coffee are stimulating, and although tea has a relatively lower level of caffeine than coffee it is likely that you will have one pot rather than one cup of tea. Recently caffeine laced soft drinks have become popular and these combine the stimulant effect of caffeine with a high glucose content – this combination can be particularly hard on the system. These drinks are often used by individuals looking for an energy boost before a session of exercise, but this influences the body into producing and consuming far more energy than it normally would. This extra energy comes at a high price, the cost being a more or less permanent depletion of vital resources; you could look at it as borrowing tomorrow's energy for today.

Any food or drink that contains physiologically active substances, apart from normal nutrients and materials essential to bodily maintenance and function, may be comparatively harmless when it is consumed merely for its enjoyable flavour and in moderate amounts. It is unlikely in this situation to produce any true addiction. But if the person becomes aware of the energy promoting, pain-relieving, anxiety-reducing or tension-relaxing effect of any particular substance and starts to *need* it then there is the potential for real dependency. If these dangers are not recognised, and no steps taken to re-establish a more balanced approach, then there is a real likelihood that the dependency can develop to the point of true addiction.

Interestingly, there is a similar danger with certain foods that most people would not immediately think of as resembling drugs in any way. Everyday examples are rhubarb, prunes and figs, which for a fair proportion of individuals have a noticeably laxative effect. If such foods are eaten simply because they are pleasant, and no obvious disturbance to bowel rhythm occurs, they are harmless nutrients, but if they are taken *because* they make the bowels move they are – for that person at least – medication. If prunes affect you in that way, the sooner you discontinue them and replace them with some equivalent dried fruit which has no physiologically disturbing property, the better your chances of maintaining your gut health.

LIVE WELL. EAT WELL. BE WELL.

Toughness

Another aspect of vital capacity is the overall integrity and toughness of your body. To be strong and resilient materials must combine tensile strength and an ability to absorb stress. Relating this to your body, the sheer strength of your physical makeup is one aspect of toughness or vital capacity. Equally important is our ability to deal with stress, to be adaptable. It is in this second factor that so many of us find ourselves lacking. We 'take things badly', harbour grudges, feel hurt or indulge in envy or hate. Instead of adapting ourselves to any unwelcome change of circumstances, we develop a state of resentment and emotional tension.

An engineer would say that the energy of stress produces strain in a material. This means that when enough pressure is applied (stress), the subject alters detectably in shape (strain). In human terms, when the load upon us becomes abnormally heavy, we should alter our 'shape', meaning not necessarily our visible form, but also our personality, the way we react to things. The alteration need not be major. Just as with metals, an almost imperceptible change in shape can absorb a great deal of energy and so avoid a total fracture. By giving way just a tiny bit we also can avoid being seriously damaged, whereas if we adopt a totally uncompromising attitude, a sufficiently powerful stress can break us.

Repairability

Once broken a structure cannot normally be completely restored to its original form and state, but a structure that has absorbed the excess stress by bending a little can usually be fully repaired comparatively easily. The parallel with human life is close, and we should aim to be neither brittle steel nor totally yielding lead. We should try to be well tempered, able to absorb the normal shocks of life without injury. By giving way elastically we can spring back to our characteristic form and resume our normal shape after being affected by an excessive impact. A slightly bowed human being has every prospect of being restored by the powerful self-healing forces in their own body, but a shattered personality presents an infinitely greater problem.

Another engineering fact regards the potential weakness of homogeneous materials that are without inconsistencies of character and without weaknesses. These must fail completely when a stress produces even the tiniest crack. Take as an example diamond, made of carbon and the hardest natural substance known. Diamond is incredibly strong and durable, but a blow that catches it on a cleavage plane will easily break it apart. By contrast, materials with inconsistencies in their makeup can be grossly overstrained without total collapse. Wrought iron is an impure material, and its very impurity gives it toughness. When over-stressed, a microscopic section breaks apart, and in doing so absorbs the energy of the stress. The fracture travels no further than the microscopically adjacent, but different, particle. The energy of the impact is absorbed with very little detriment to the total strength and appearance of the structure.

Dangerous idealism

We could draw parallels almost limitlessly, but for the moment it is enough to underline one message: for a human being to be tough they must be resilient and just a little bit inconsistent – they must have a few honest human weaknesses. Being genuinely tough means having the ability to be battered by the world without completely losing your own character. To succeed in being utterly consistent is to make yourself dangerously vulnerable; it is putting all your eggs in one basket. For instance, the more highly an individual is educated in a particular field, and the more completely they allow a narrow idealism to dominate their life, the further they move into this fragile category. A jack-of-all-trades has a broader range of interests and abilities and therefore more options if one of their skills is threatened.

And a final point from the engineers: A metal which can withstand attack from a particular chemical indefinitely, or which can support a given physical stress without yielding, quickly breaks when the two stresses are combined. So when a human body breaks down, it is almost never from a single cause; in nearly every case, there is a combination of stresses, of different kinds, operating against different aspects of the individual's system.

Most humans can stand up to an atrocious physical environment, or to cruel and intense emotional distress, or to sub-standard nutritional resources, but combine any two and their prospects are dramatically diminished. Subject an individual to all three, and those prospects dwindle to almost zero. The relationship of physical toughness to vital capacity is clear enough. Emotional toughness in all its forms; morale, confidence, resourcefulness, is just as significant. But a person who can tolerate acute pain, caused by something they believe deeply in, will collapse distressingly when doubt consumes them. Not only do they become unable to bear the pain, but their physical body also gives way under stresses that it previously withstood easily.

Faith

Confidence in the day-to-day activities of your body is an essential part of good vital capacity. Many people have no faith whatsoever in their body's ability to cope with common disorders, largely because they have been told from an early age to regard acute illnesses as damaging attacks which must be stopped. The vital capacity of an individual can be undermined by the credence they place upon the negative messages offered by medical doctors, the big pharmaceutical companies and even by the vendors of alternative remedies.

So there is no way of increasing your vital capacity and this might sound like a discouraging and pessimistic view but that is not the intention. Our aim is to stress that a realistic approach can lead to constructive action; hope of finding a miraculous solution to your problems will almost invariably be unproductive and disappointing.

Making the best possible use of your resources is an approach that cannot be improved upon. Living on comforting but mistaken beliefs can lead to premature deterioration, and ultimately premature death, whereas acceptance of an uncomfortable truth may lead – via an equally uncomfortable road initially – to an extended and more effective life. Recognising your limitations is not surrender, it is the acceptance of a challenge.

LIVE WELL. EAT WELL. BE WELL.

Points to remember

1 All life depends upon vitality, but vitality is not elastic nor it is a purchasable commodity, you cannot buy more if you run out.

2 *Vitality* is not the same thing as *energy*.

3 Vitality cannot be restored once it has been consumed.

4 If the vitality of the individual is well matched to their energy, you have a balanced individual.

5 Vitality is consumed in many ways, often insidiously.

6 The longer and the more completely we live simply and sensibly according to the inescapable rules of our physical existence; the more fully and effectively our bodies will co-operate and be in harmony with our conscious selves.

7 In our late fifties and early sixties most of us will notice reduced levels of vitality, this is normal in all but the most excellent physical specimens. Learn to work within your limitations.

8 When vitality wanes an increasing dependence upon stimulants often increases. Extra cups of tea or coffee or energy drinks become the norm and we start to use up tomorrow's energy today.

9 When the individual feels a need for a particular food or drink, they have become hooked. In current terminology, they are not an addict, but 'dependent'. This may sound far-fetched but it changes our relationship with our everyday nutrition.

10 A human being can stand up to an atrocious physical environment, or to cruel and intense emotional distress, or to sub-standard nutritional resources; but combine any two and their prospects are dramatically diminished: subject an individual to all three, and those prospects dwindle to become almost zero.

11 Confidence in the somatic sense and intelligence of one's body is an essential part of good vital capacity.

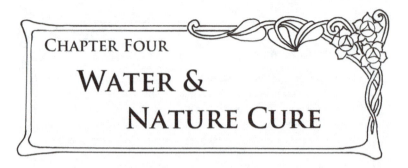

CHAPTER FOUR
WATER &
NATURE CURE

With advice on home treatment

THE USE OF water in a therapeutic way has always been a part of the Nature Cure teachings. Hydrotherapy has a long and sometimes complex history, and we certainly don't embrace the more extreme treatments beloved of the early proponents. But out of their early practice and applications some of the essential principles and practice of the use of water in natural healing have evolved.

As time went on hydrotherapists, or water curers, gradually tempered their treatments and started to combine these with sensible feeding and exercise regimes, this resulted in some excellent, lasting results. Soon, patients who had been declared incurable by orthodox methods began to seek and receive help from hydropathic teachers. The movement inevitably developed in several different ways, one of which was through Dr Henry Lindlahr Nature Cure School in Illinois, USA. The methods and treatments still used are directly descended from Lindlahr work and have been further refined through the extensive clinical experience of my grandfather, grandmother, father and uncle at the Kingston Clinic.

The great thing about the simplified versions of the early practices is that they can easily be achieved at home and with materials that are usually readily to hand. This meant that patients were able to continue the applications that were so usefully employed during their stay in the clinic without having to buy any costly equipment.

Sweat

Elsewhere in the world, water-treatment continued to be used, although often based on different theories and understanding. In the Northern Hemisphere the preference was for some form of intense overheating before applying cold water. The sauna, followed by the cold immersion, has a profound effect on the individual. Often an interruption of any immediate symptoms was offered as proof of the effectiveness of the process. While this method may have no ill effect on those of fair vitality, and may produce some beneficial activity in a skin which otherwise has had too little stimulation, there are potential dangers for a less than vital person trying to regain health. The useful elimination of wastes through the skin is not proportional to the amount of sweat, and the expenditure of bodily energy can be more enervating than effective.

Of all the characteristics of sweat-baths, the most misleading is probably the appearance of vigorous perspiration. This is usually taken as clear evidence of benefit. More truthfully, the production of copious sweat is likely to be a sign of distress, not of vigorous health. To be truly effective as a cooling mechanism, perspiration should evaporate as soon as it reaches the surface of the skin. In this way it absorbs a great deal of heat from the skin, it also helps to cool the blood flowing immediately below the surface. It is one of the ways your body maintains homeostasis or internal balance.

So sweat that lies on or trickles over your skin in droplets does not appreciably lower your body's temperature; it merely makes you more uncomfortable. If your body is producing profuse perspiration it is more likely to be an attempt to avoid overheating and is almost always a sign of vital strain.

Salt

The claimed benefits from the copious sweating induced by the baths as a means of eliminating wastes freely are true to a point, but ultimately this method can often prove to be disappointing. Tests have shown that the sweat produced for the first few minutes in a sauna or similar has a high proportion of waste content, but thereafter it consists almost entirely of water and essential salts. Of course ejecting toxic waste in the form of harmful trace elements must be helpful, but the loss of essential and beneficial salts is not. Any efforts to replace lost salts with salty foods and lost fluid with an increased intake of water is not ideal. The salt in processed foods is not the same as the salts in the balanced form found in organic whole fruits, salads and vegetables. It is sodium chloride and it is more likely to make your body retain the water that you are now taking to excess to replace the fluids lost through excessive sweating. The tendency, therefore, is for your body to become depleted in essential organised minerals as well as to retain fluids.

However, the massaging and the cold applications which normally form part of a Turkish bath can go a long way to improving the vitality of your skin. It can also encourage more vigorous function of this our largest organ for some days afterwards. Luckily, we are sure that just as effective results can be produced by simpler methods, without involving any vital strain or apparatus.

Responses to heat and cold

Generally, heat applied to your skin has no lastingly beneficial effect on your system as a whole. For a comparatively short time it can be very soothing and can, for instance, take the pain out of an aching joint. But we tend to extend the application so that nerves become numbed, your circulation slows and your body's own heat-production is depressed. The internal temperature of the body is controlled within close limits, and the mechanism is quickly and powerfully influenced by the temperature of the skin. When the surface is chilled, heat-production is automatically increased in anticipation of continued loss of warmth through the skin. Conversely, if the skin is heated combustion is suppressed in order to avoid any risk of internal overheating.

When you apply cold water to the skin in the right way, the effects are almost exactly the reverse. Your internal heat-production response is initiated and, after a series of reactions, the circulation of the blood is made freer and more effective. One result is that injured skin and sub-cutaneous tissues are more able to start essential repair work. However, it must be clearly understood that cold itself does not speed up any vital activity. The real benefit comes from the internally produced warmth and increased activity, which the application of the cold compress induces in a normally responding system.

When you apply cold water the first effect is to cool the skin, and this drives the blood away from the surface by causing the nerves there to constrict the blood vessels. This is your body's natural defence mechanism: by withdrawing the blood from the skin's surface there is less risk of loss of heat from the body. It is possible to override this reaction by drinking alcohol, which will cause the surface blood vessels, the capillaries, to dilate and produce a warm glow to your skin. But this response is at the expense of your internal temperature balance. This is why we don't recommend alcohol when you have been exposed to extreme cold.

Care must be taken with the application of cold water in any form, and just as with heat prolonged over-exposure should be avoided. If the cold application is too extreme, as in the use of ice packs, or is continued for too long by immersing in really cold water – the vessels on the surface of your skin may remain constricted. Your skin will tend to go pale and may even become bluish, despite the fact that your body, as a whole, is striving to produce more heat to restore normal circulation. There is a limit to what your system can do, and if the external cold application is maintained for too long the surface flesh can suffer. As an illustration; you can see the results in relatively mild cases as chilblains, and in the more extreme cases as frostbite.

Understanding

The forms of water treatment used in Nature Cure practice involve application of cold for a relatively short duration, with a few specialised exceptions application time is a matter of only seconds or minutes. The whole aim is to assist your body's functions, not to obstruct or numb them. The cold is intended to produce a warm, active response. With such brief applications, the colder the water is when applied, the better the warm reaction will be. It is this reaction which we see as the essence of effective hydrotherapy, and the more drastic the situation is perceived by your body the more vigorously it will attempt to compensate.

However, because of the strength of the reaction, care and understanding are essential when deciding on and administering water treatment. A trained Nature Cure practitioner will make some preliminary estimates of your body's fitness. It is as ineffective to take half-measures with a really vital subject as it is potentially dangerous to over-chill someone who is unwell. When in doubt a practitioner will err on the side of caution, and it usually becomes obvious very quickly what you and your body can handle most effectively and comfortably. The drastic remedies that were so much a part of early hydrotherapy a century ago are not a part of the Nature Cure philosophy. We prefer the principle that the more seriously ill the patient, the more imperative it is to avoid any violence in treatment. There will be more information later about individual applications, as well as more detailed descriptions of various useful techniques that you can apply at home.

In some forms of water-treatment the water has no particular significance other than its easy availability and its huge variability in temperature. That is, any other fluid would be almost as effective in cooling or warming the skin; but water has three considerable and outstanding virtues: it is clean, it is non-poisonous and it absorbs a lot of heat in the process of becoming warmed. In other forms of treatment, the water takes a much more active part and in this its characteristics are even more vital. It provides an atmosphere which seems ideal for the rapid repair of injury and which makes easy the ejection of dirt and other foreign matter that would otherwise complicate the healing of a wound. It allows surface damage to heal with a minimum of scarring by keeping the tissues soft and permeable to the nutrient and scavenging constituents of the bloodstream.

This contrasts strongly with what happens when external injuries are treated with antiseptics, which far from aiding healing can considerably delay recovery and increase scarring. This occurs partly through the additional injury that the chemical inflicts on tissue, thereby increasing the actual numbers of damaged and destroyed cells involved, and partly by drying and hardening the flesh so that repair activity is slowed and obstructed. Our domesticated animals can give us a lesson here; a dog with a wound will lick it continually. No matter how unwholesome the creature's feeding, its saliva is infinitely more helpful to healing than any man-made antiseptic.

Why no equipment?

If you already know a bit about water treatments you might be familiar with some of their many forms. Douches and sprays of all sizes, directions and pressures have been used, as have prolonged immersions in sitz baths, wetted cloths of varying sizes in packs and compresses, and some rather more picturesque special applications, such as the 'dewy-grass walking' associated with the name of Father Sebastian Kneipp, to name but a few.

When my grandfather opened his first clinic in Edinburgh in 1912 he had quite a collection of equipment for water treatments, but over the decades he dismantled and discarded the expensive array of pressure gauges, temperature meters, regulating valves, nozzles, jets, sprays, sitz baths and cabinets which were once so busily employed. Possibly the strongest argument for this was the realisation that whenever apparatus of any kind is used in treatment, the patient tends to regard the machine as having the curative powers. No matter how hard he tried to explain otherwise, the person undergoing mechanised treatment inevitably feels that the apparatus must be playing a vital part.

Even if the device by which water is applied is not of a mechanical nature, but something quite natural – such as peat, mud or even dung – it is only human nature to credit the inanimate and inactive container or applicator with greater value than the true reagents – the water itself and the response of your own body to that water. We are quite confident that clean cloths are preferable to any mucky but water-absorbing materials, and at least as effective; yet there are many people who cheerfully pay pounds for a mud-pack and yet refuse to apply an almost cost free cold water waist compress.

Selling merchandise is not part of our work; our aim is essentially to teach you how to live healthily. We prefer to persuade those of you who have lost your self-confidence that your fears are unfounded; and we explore this aspect of our approach in the chapter on The Fear Factor. With the right support, and logical approaches and lifestyle changes, your morale and physique can be restored. The Nature Cure practitioners' task is to demonstrate to you ways that mean you can help yourself to regain normal function, and ultimately persuade you not to rely indefinitely on our assistance. Accordingly, our ultimate aim is to bring treatment of all types to its least complicated and most direct form. This means eliminating all disguise and ornamentation – no matter how harmless and innocent these may seem – so that it is the substance, not the trimmings, which is important. If you have become accustomed to having to purchase something to achieve a cure, our methods may seem less immediately effective. You might feel that we are giving less than you had been led to expect. So we had better explain the processes in some detail.

With any properly designed apparatus it is usually possible to carry out a given operation with greater efficiency and with less human effort than by unaided manual exertion: this is true as much in hydrotherapy as in any other activity. With gauges and regulators it is possible to give a more accurately controlled douche, spray or immersion than without them. But unless you continue to receive professional assistance, or buy expensive apparatus for your own use, the application of the treatment is inevitably limited. As soon as you leave the hydropathic establishment, you are cut off from the seemingly essential gadgetry. Unable to continue with the mechanised treatment, you find those helpful water applications a rapidly fading memory.

Compare this with the simpler option, in which all the materials and equipment you need can be found in any ordinary household. In this case, you will quickly learn to apply these either alone or with a minimum of help, and with little discomfort or effort. There is not the slightest need to break your newly acquired routines and once established it will be easier to keep up the water treatments than to forget them. The plain truth is that in matters of human health a perfect system of treatment for three weeks, or three months, is in the long run less effective than a simpler and less exacting routine lived with through time.

What this means is that one or two simple water exercises can become part of an easy set of daily habits. Other slightly more elaborate hydropathic applications can be kept in reserve; to be confidently practised when systemic spring-cleanings such as a 'healing crises' or when accidental injuries occur. Another factor in our deliberate simplification and domestication of hydrotherapy is that we do not regard it as a complete system in itself.

Cold water

Dr Henry Lindlahr, known affectionately as the father of modern Nature Cure, has recognised the value of hydrotherapy but he also recognised its limitations. His estimate is well summarised in his own words, 'There is no such thing as a cure-all; but if there were, it would be cold water, properly applied.'

It is vital to omit no part of that summary; every word is

significant and any attempt to simplify the sentence can completely invert its meaning and sense.

Let us now turn to more practical aspects of hydrotherapy, and look at the details of some everyday water applications and a few emergency treatments.

Compresses

The Cold Compress, or Wet Pack, is an essential part of any Nature Cure follower's everyday gear. The names are a little unfortunate, suggesting a miserable cold clamminess, whereas the reality is a glowing and relaxing comfort, giving rapid relief from many forms of distress. However, the cold compress must be correctly applied to produce a normal response, so an explanation of the basic functions and purposes is essential. A misapplied compress can fail utterly, and may even do harm, so if you are a novice it is really important, initially, only to use the compress as and when directed by your practitioner. Within a short time, you will learn enough to be able to decide when further applications are desirable, or when they should be discontinued. However, please beware of becoming evangelical about compresses, because it is easy to imagine that what works for you must produce a similar effect in everyone else. Although the chances may be reasonable, there is still enough possibility of a totally different reaction to make any indiscriminate recommendation to your friends unwise.

The main function of a compress is to produce moist warmth on the chosen area of the body over a period of several hours. As already noted, moist warmth presents the ideal condition for healing activity, and it is essential that the warmth should come from your own body. This is most likely to occur when the compress applied is really cold; far from being a kindness, a tepid compress usually fails to produce a good response and you can easily become chilled and depressed instead of experiencing a warm glow. It is equally a mistake to try to 'help' a compress by holding a hot-water-bottle against it. A note of caution here: if you are unable to react with normal vigour to the compress, and it fails to warm up within a few minutes, it means that there is either too great a volume of water in it, or that you are in a state of depressed vitality and this contraindicates its use. Heroic perseverance is totally out of place here and can easily be counterproductive.

How to make and apply a cold compress

The compress consists of two parts: Part one is a piece of thin cotton or linen cloth, a scrap of old sheeting or shirting is suitable (N.B. It should be pure cotton, not poly-cotton and preferably not dyed or printed) and part two is a larger strip of woollen material, preferably knitted or loosely woven. For the most commonly used form – the waist compress – the thin cloth should be between five and ten inches wide – depending on your body size – and long enough to go round the waist with a couple of inches of overlap. The woollen material should be a bit broader, and long enough to go round at least twice: a large knitted scarf is ideal, with its natural elasticity, but failing this a strip of woollen blanketing will serve (provided that it does not cause itching or discomfort). The thin material is soaked in cold water, squeezed out firmly so that it no longer drips, and placed directly on the skin. The dry woollen material is wrapped around over it, and fastened firmly with one or two safety pins. The wool should be tight enough to stay securely in place, but not so constricting as to interfere with your breathing. It is important that the woollen material should be all wool, since any mixture with other fibres can make it absorbent

HOW TO APPLY A COLD WATER COMPRESS

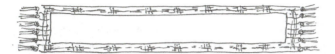

Take a long woollen scarf and lay it out on your bed. If it is long enough, fold it into two layers. Take a strip of cotton 4-5 inches wide and long enough to go round your middle. Soak it in cold water and wring it out until it no longer drips. Lay it on top of the woollen scarf.

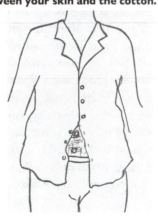

Stand with your back to the bed and grasp the scarf and cotton strip together, quickly wrap it around your middle. Remember to tuck your top out of the way so it doesn't end up between your skin and the cotton.

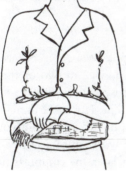

Secure the layers with a large safety pin and pull down your top to cover the compress. Get into bed immediately. The compress should warm up in less than 5 minutes. This is important - if it remains cold take it off and try again in about half an hour. If this also fails take it off and leave it off.

and the heat-retention properties are reduced. In case of doubt, be generous with the woollen covering, both as to width and as to the number of layers applied.

You will eventually devise your own pet method of putting on your waist compress quickly and easily, but the following may be a useful starting point: lay the woollen material flat out along the edge of the bed and lay the damp cloth on top, then turn your back to the compress, pick up the two layers together at the ends and bring them to the body in a single movement. This brings the ends of the cloth to the front, where they may be easily adjusted, and it can all be achieved in a matter of one or two seconds. A variant is to lay the cloths, in the same sequence, but across the bed, and then to lie down on them and pull over the ends to fasten them.

Variations

After the first mild shock of the cold application, the compress should begin to warm up. This should happen in two or three minutes, and it usually becomes quite cosy within three to five minutes. If you experience feelings of chilliness for more than five minutes the compress should be taken off, put aside, and your skin dried. After allowing your body to work up to a normally warm state, usually around half an hour later, the compress can be reapplied. In most cases, this is quite effective, the repeated brief cooling producing a vigorous response and active circulation, so that the second time around the compress warms up quite quickly. However, if you are still not experiencing a ready reaction you should take the compress off and leave it off. On the next occasion, it will probably be more effective to reduce the width of the damp material by half, or to use a thinner piece of cloth in order to coax your body into a better response.

It is most usual to apply the waist compress overnight, or you can use one throughout the day if you are unwell and are staying in bed. Either way it is important to get into bed immediately and under the covers. Any delay in getting under the bedclothes, even sitting up in bed to read, can cause chilling and prevent the normal beneficial warm reaction.

The Body Compress is of similar form to the waist compress, but considerably broader. It can be up to 18 inches wide and it extends from under the arms to over the hips. You would usually use a body compress in conditions where heat production is no problem, typically, if you are in a feverish state, or to soothe the skin-rash conditions of childhood. It should be noted, however, that the intention of such a compress is not 'to bring down the fever'. Although the application may give you very welcome relief, the amount of cold water in a compress is quite negligible by comparison with the mass of your body. The effect is totally different from that of an ice pack or an extended cold bath, both of which can chill you down with possibly serious results. The compress does not obstruct your body's processes; rather it removes the tensions that could obstruct them, and so allows the vital functions of the fever or rash to be completed in a less distressing way.

For the neck – a region where tensions are commonly found – a compress is essentially the same as one for the waist, scaled down suitably. In most households, handy materials are a large handkerchief folded twice in the same direction, to make a narrow strip, and a woollen sock applied over the top. If you apply a neck compress it is wise to also put on a waist compress to balance the reaction and avoid too much activity being centred on your neck. This is an important point and will be explained more fully later.

Vital sleep

The most noticeable effect of a compress is an increase in the volume and flow of the blood circulation in the tissues it covers. We have mentioned the process of reaction that causes the blood vessels near the surface to dilate, and operating through the nervous controls a similar relaxation of more deeply situated vessels can also occur. A waist compress worn at night usually makes deeper and more restful sleep possible, although not necessarily longer sleep, rather a feeling of greater refreshment on waking. Vital organs lying under the surface are also influenced: in many cases your kidneys show this by producing urine in greater quantity or with a higher concentration of wastes. Your liver and lungs may be similarly encouraged in their work, with corresponding benefit to the condition of your blood.

More superficially, the sweat glands of your skin are activated and a vigorous elimination of watery and gaseous wastes happens. It is quite possible for these wastes to be sufficiently acidic to irritate your skin and produce a rash. There is nothing dangerous about this 'compress rash', it will subside by discontinuing the application for a night or two, but if it is misunderstood and treated with suppressive salves or other medication, there could be counterproductive outcomes. Just give your body the time it needs to settle down at its own pace.

If you are only using a waist compress, the increased flow of wastes through your skin can be merely uncomfortable; but if the compress is applied over more delicate parts of your body such as the throat, eyes or ears great caution should be exercised. The tissues in these parts of your body may not be able to handle the extra traffic without injury or distress. We recommend that such localised areas should only be compressed with professional guidance. Even a foot or a hand may, if your bloodstream is more waste-laden than usual, develop a distressing concentration of activity if treated with only a local compress. Always balance a substantial compress on any other part of the body with a waist compress at night or when in bed.

Unusual effects

Occasionally, the acidic wastes emerging through your skin are concentrated enough, or of such a composition, that your compress material falls apart after only a few applications. Certain types of waste may cause discolouration or even bright staining of the cloth, often as a result of your having taken certain drugs in the past. The elimination of these toxic materials rarely causes any discomfort, but it is important to wash the skin after removing the compress. The inner cloth of the compress should be washed thoroughly in hot, soapy water daily, and boiled at least once per week if you are using it regularly.

The four important conditions about the use of compresses have already been mentioned but it might be useful to reiterate them:

1 In the early stages at least, use no more than a single layer of thin, damp material, well wrung out; but be generous with the woollen covering.

2 Unless under experienced guidance, do not apply a compress to the neck or to any part of the head.

3 Any local compress (such as on fingers, knee, eye or ear) is liable to stir up local activity to an uncomfortable degree, unless accompanied by a waist compress. (A compress on an injured hand may be worn 24 hours a day, so long as a waist compress is used each night.) For this reason, it is

useful to be familiar with the waist compress, and to be able to react well to it, before attempting local applications.

4   Resist the charitable impulse to advise your friends about compresses. Uninformed prescription is likely to be ineffective, and in certain cases could be harmful.

Squat Splash

The Squat Splash is probably the most widely recommended and most often used form of everyday water applications. In its simplest form it combines the beneficial effects of such specialised hydropathic techniques as the Perineal Douche, the Genito-Urinary Spray and the Sitz Bath without requiring the relatively complex equipment associated with these. It is best applied in the morning, preferably following a short spell of exercise, and after emptying the bladder and possibly the bowels as well. It is also an effective follow-up to exercises later in the day, especially those directed to improving the state of your abdomen and its muscles.

To have a Squat Splash run three to four inches of cold water into your bath, this should be as cold as possible and certainly not 'tempered' by adding any hot water, and squat in the bath with only your toes immersed. With the hands, generous scoops of water are then thrown up onto your body, alternately aimed at the lower part of the abdomen and at the perineum (the pelvic floor). The splashes should be applied in a slow, steady rhythm, so that each causes a vigorous contraction of the muscles, but the entire bath should not last for more than about half a minute. Much longer applications tend to lose effectiveness, whereas if the water is really cold – not over 45° F. (7° C.) – half a dozen splashes may produce an excellent response. The bathroom should be comfortably warm, but if it is not, the splash can be applied without undressing completely. One hand is used to hold your clothing out of the way while your free hand scoops up the water.

An alternative to the Squat Splash is to use a showerhead on a flexible hose. The water should be cold – with no adding of hot water – and of reasonable strength of flow, the spray can be directed at the same areas that the Squat Splash reaches and is usually just as effective. A specifically directed flow of cold water will give a good response with 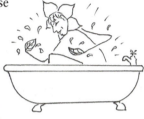 less chilling and the purely thermal effect of the cold water is intensified by the mechanical activity. You might be more comfortable using your hands to apply the water to your chest and neck areas. Here again, however, the aim should be to produce the best response, not to extend the cold application unduly. With a shower, one small point is worth attention: for most people it is preferable to take the first impact of the cold water on the lower part of the body, and then if comfortable apply to the chest. If the chest is sprayed first there may be an unpleasant constriction of heart and lungs.

Basically, you will evolve a simple and straightforward cold splash routine that best suits you and your lifestyle, and once you get into the habit you will find it a very refreshing start to your day.

Abdominal tone

The effects of the Squat Splash, or the pelvic application of your cold shower, can be particularly noticeable on your abdominal wall. Congestion, as is often found in someone with weak abdominal muscles is usually improved quite quickly, as will be the general tone of your abdominal muscles. If you can also carry out some simple exercises for the abdomen before your cold splash or shower, and also make an effort to draw your tummy up from within while splashing, there should be a marked sensation of a bracing and warm glow throughout afterwards.

Some people like to follow their Squat Splash with an overall immersion. While this is perfectly good for a reasonably fit person, it can too easily dissipate the effect and lessen the remedial function if your pelvic and abdominal structures are in a devitalised state.

The Squat Splash is a valuable follow-up to the specialised exercises that we recommend in cases of haemorrhoids, prolapse and other conditions of pelvic distress. However, it is important that you take advice and guidance from an experienced Nature Cure practitioner before attempting any of the techniques. A cold application can seriously aggravate your condition when the structures are out of their proper position.

Another aspect of the Squat Splash, or Pelvic Shower, is that it is an effective substitute for the bidet. In this country, the bidet is still regarded as a rather comic rarity, and even those who would like to equip their bathrooms with it are liable to be discouraged by the expensive installation that our plumbing regulations demand. For those with fairly regular and predictable bowel action, it is simple to make a routine of a Squat Splash immediately following.

'Hundred up'

Running on the spot is a more easily achieved equivalent of Father Kneipp's dewy grass walking, and is more practical for most town-dwellers. It can be gentle or strenuous, as desired, and requires the same amount of cold water in the bath as the Squat Splash – which it may well precede. The movement is just what it sounds like – stamping quickly with alternate feet in the cold water. It can initially be rather an untidy activity, but experience in controlling your feet can usually minimise the showering of the bathroom.

The effect is, once again, principally due to the nervous reactions. The soles of the feet are richly supplied with sensitive nerve endings (if you wish confirmation, ask a friend to tickle your soles), and the tonic effect improves the condition of the entire foot. The benefit is particularly noticeable with flat foot – fallen arches – especially if an effort is made to hold the instep high and with the big toe curled inward, so that the outer edge of the foot takes the weight. However, it is not only the foot which benefits from the cold stamp; there is a powerful nervous linkage between the feet and the lower area of the abdomen and back. There are practitioners of reflexology who devote almost their entire attention to the feet, asserting that they are able to induce 'cures' in any part of the system solely by manipulations of the feet. While we regard this as an exaggerated claim based on a philosophy different from our own, there can be no denial of the fact that pelvic tone and the condition of the feet are closely linked, so that if anything is done to improve one, the other tends to benefit correspondingly.

Three-second plunge

The total-immersion, or three second plunge, cold bath, as a morning routine, is traditionally symbolic of really serious health seeking. Yet we rarely recommend it to our patients. This is not because we are becoming soft-hearted, but because we have found in most cases a reaction that is just as effective can be produced by other, less drastic, methods. The methods we prefer are also less daunting to the newcomer and far less likely to cause chilling. It is true that, when properly applied, the actual chilling effect of a cold bath should be quite moderate, but for many people a cold bath is equated to a form of punishment. They picture themselves remaining immersed until they feel really cold and miserable, instead of seeing how quickly they can get in, do the business, and get out. There is no benefit to chilling your system, and the real purpose of a cold bath, or any cold splash or shower, is to increase vital activity. This improved vital activity is indicated by the experience of increased warmth that characterises a good reaction. Be under no illusion, if no warm response is produced then the bath is fundamentally a failure. To ensure a good reaction, an important aspect is the skin rub immediately after the immersion. Some prefer an extra-rough towel, while others prefer really vigorous rubbing of the skin, until quite dry, with the hands alone. Whichever method you prefer the room that you use should be reasonably warm.

The hand rub

The hand rub is a somewhat modified form of the overall cold bath, and is often preferable to total, or even partial, immersion. Dip your hands in cold water and rub them over your whole body, with additional dipping as required. This method causes far less chilling than the total plunge, yet because of the vigorous activity it is capable of producing quite an effective reaction.

Use of water in emergency situations

Up to now we have been concerned mainly with routine forms of water application, but the historical appreciation of water rests much more heavily on its value in emergencies. In a sense, this is the more instinctive use, since it does not depend on reasoning or even on observation and often time is of the essence.

Cuts and burns

Water-treatment is appropriate in all manner of minor cuts, burns and similar injuries. It is also effective in more severe injuries, although with these there may be the complication of necessary surgical attention before water can be usefully applied. Much depends on your confidence that water-treatment alone is adequate for the degree of injury. Certainly if you feel a real need for surgical attention, it is not for any well-meaning bystander, or Nature Cure practitioner, to oppose it. Conversely, if you have the confidence, seemingly miraculous recoveries can occur without any form of surgical attention. We all know that it is in emergencies that the true character of an individual shows up, and this is certainly true in the case of personal injuries. So many factors may be involved that only the most generalised advice can be offered here, and only through experience can you begin to lose your doubts and become more confident in your body's own healing capabilities.

Simple surface cuts offer possibly the most dramatic proof of the efficacy of water-treatment. They were probably the first conditions to be treated in this way, since every land animal seems to know instinctively that a cut should be kept moist, either by licking or by wading in a stream. Silesian farmer Vincent Priessnitz began his practice some 200 years ago by applying water to various ailing and injured domestic animals. It was from these early treatments that he acquired a reputation among neighbouring farmers, who called him to heal their beasts. From animals, he went on to practise on himself, after being forced to do so as the result of an accident that his medical advisers were unable to treat. Although his injuries were largely internal, he found that water applications had a beneficial effect below the surface. Indeed, the only difference is that with a superficial injury anyone may see for himself how clean and rapid the healing can be with proper water-treatment. That similar treatment produces conditions favourable to speedy and effective internal healing calls for a little more self-belief and a chance to experience it for yourself.

Cleanliness

The important necessity is to keep the wound damp until it has completely healed, that is, until the skin has reformed into an unbroken surface. This allows the damaged tissues to eject without difficulty any dirt that may have been carried into the wound. It also keeps the injured surfaces in the soft condition that allows healing – 'granulation' – to proceed rapidly and with a minimum of eventual scarring. Scab formation is almost negligible, pus oozes painlessly out and the formation of deep, sealed-off pockets is almost impossible.

In the water-treatment of any wound, three points should be observed:

1   The bandage should not be so tight as to interfere with the free circulation of the blood in the region.
2   There should be no waterproof layer – which would either prevent the free access of air or the escape of fluid or gaseous wastes.
3   The injured area should not be allowed to attract wastes from the body as a whole. This is liable to occur in an individual with heavy accumulations of toxins throughout their system and in the bloodstream.
4   Apply a waist compress at night to assist your body to deal with the repair work.

The first two of these points are obvious enough, but the third calls for explanation. Dr Henry Lindlahr called the situation 'The

Fontanelle Effect', and it goes some way to explain why some people develop what is called 'blood poisoning' from seemingly slight scratches. Of course, in some cases, it is possible that highly toxic material from the outside have poisoned the skin and subcutaneous tissues, but in the majority of badly inflamed wounds the toxins do not come from outside but from inside the body. The comparatively minor inflammation set up by the injury attracts a concentration of wastes from the blood-stream, and if there is already a small flow of escaping wastes from the injured tissues, this tends to be greatly augmented. A compress worn over any small area of the body encourages just such direct elimination and, in an unhealthy body, the resultant activity may cause more than discomfort: it can produce quite serious destruction of the flesh around the original wound. This sequence accounts also for the advice given earlier about taking great care when using local compresses, and to avoid areas away from the cleansing organs that are normally equipped for waste-elimination or blood-purification. The fourth point is dealt with below.

Safeguards

Where there is the least doubt about the progress of healing, or about the general health of the individual, a waist compress should be applied at the same time as the bandage to the injury. Around the waist and upper abdomen are grouped the main blood-cleansing organs, and in addition the waist compress itself covers a comparatively large area of skin, so that the entire region is capable of handling without distress any extra work which the local compress may induce. If the wound is relatively serious, and is accompanied by a degree of shock, then the patient should lie down in a quiet warm place until the initial trauma has passed.

If you are in a reasonable state of health you should be able to safely apply a simple bandage on a cut finger or hand, and the only precaution is to keep the bandage moist and clean. However, you should also keep an eye open for any signs of excessive inflammation or excessive pus-formation. Inflammation and pus are normal accompaniments of vigorous cleaning-up of damaged tissues, but if they appear to be out of proportion to the severity of the injury, a 'Fontanelle' should be suspected.

Excessive distress also suggests that a temporary reduction of food might be helpful, particularly the cutting out of proteins, fats and sugary things. (It is a rule of thumb that pus production indicates a need to reduce protein consumption; while refined sugars are notorious for hindering healing processes.) In any case of injury, the best possible chances of clean, rapid healing happen when the smallest demands are made on your digestive tract. In serious cases a complete fast for one or two days is recommended as the treatment of choice. Along with this limiting of food intake, if you are injured you should seek peace and quiet, shock will almost certainly be a part of your body's reaction to the injury or burn, and no stimulants should be taken at this time. No cups of tea for shock, no coffee, no glucose drinks, just sips of water as required and get as much sleep and rest as you can get.

Deep cuts

In the case of a deep cut, any dirt should be washed out as completely as possible. If no water is immediately available, make the wound bleed freely for a few seconds as this can carry out material that would otherwise cause complications. However, assuming a supply of clean water, allow this to run freely into the wound for a minute or two. If there is grease in the dirt, plain soap may even be used. Prompt action is important; at this stage the wound is numbed by shock, and the cold water itself lessens the sensitivity at the same time as cleansing the injury. Even a few minutes later, pain and inflammation will make comparable cleansing much more uncomfortable. However, do not be too concerned with trying to achieve absolute cleanliness of the wound at this stage. Provided that it is properly bandaged – with cold water – and is thereafter kept damp, there will be no sealing-in of potentially dangerous foreign matter. It can be helpful to keep the wound deliberately open at the surface by inserting an edge of linen for the first few bandagings. This naturally assumes that the wound is not so extensive that it needs stitching – although here if you are confident enough in your own body's healing abilities you may find that you can successfully cope with a wound that orthodox practitioners would rather stitch. Taking a chance is often well rewarded by the absence of complications that stitching and the use of antiseptics can cause.

Burns

For simple burns, the treatment is exactly the same as for cuts. Copious washing with really cold water eases pain and minimises shock. The cold-water compress has a lastingly soothing effect, and all one has to do is keep an eye open for the possibility of a 'Fontanelle'. Just as with a cut, it may take several days for the healing to reach its most active stage, and the appearance then of greater inflammation or of pus does not necessarily indicate any deterioration.

If the burn is more than merely superficial, it is important to use only pure linen for the immediate dressing. The reason for this is that the material will almost certainly become adherent to the injured flesh. Cotton is not stable in this situation and may rot, causing added irritation. Linen, however, is more durable and may safely be left in place for several days. Indeed, its adhesion may be deliberately encouraged, so as to provide a substitute skin while the healing takes place beneath. The linen layer is treated as skin, with the normal bandaging applied over it. All with the usual proviso: keep the area damp and use bandages that allow the flow of clean air in and any gaseous wastes to escape.

Sprains and pains

Sprains – whether of ankle, wrist or ribs – lose a lot of their agony when promptly treated with water. A powerful assistance to the blood circulation is needed, as the blood tends to be obstructed by the swelling and pressure that follow the injury. A simple cold compress will give some assistance, but alternating applications of hot and cold water can induce more immediate and positive pumping of the blood. Depending on the site of the injury and available equipment these applications may be with basins or with cloths. The mechanism is that the hot application produces a nervous relaxation of the blood vessels, which fill with blood. When the cold is then substituted, the same nervous controls constrict the vessels, and the blood is forced onward. This response is due to the presence of numerous one-way valves in the veins. By repeating the changes a large number of times – say between 10 and 20 of half a minute each – a complete and rapid renewal of blood is produced in the injured part. Also, the extremes of hot and cold tend to tire out the sensory nerves so that pain is less acutely felt. Some prefer different lengths of application for the hot and cold with the hot being less than half the time of the cold, others advise the same time period for each. Either way, the cold

LIVE WELL. EAT WELL. BE WELL.

water should be as cold as you can get and the hot as hot as you can stand. Have a kettle and ice cubes to hand to maintain temperatures. Also, as you gain more confidence in applying your own treatments you will learn which length of application suits you best.

The tolerance to heat rises as the treatment proceeds, so that small amounts of boiling water can be added to the hot bowl between each application. The cloth will remove some of the heat and the hotter water will be needed to keep the temperature up. For an ankle or wrist, bowls or basins are most convenient, but where ribs, shoulder or neck have to be treated, small towels folded into thick pads are suitable. It is important to start with hot and finish with cold – just as you'd normally say 'hot and cold' – and after the 15 minutes or so of active alternations, a cold water compress may be applied with benefit. With a severe sprain there will be shock, so missing a meal or two will not come amiss. Always remember to drink some water, especially if you are in the habit of getting most of your liquid intake from the fresh foods in your diet.

In the case of an ankle sprained far from a hot water supply, frequent immersions in cold water, tight bandaging – even with a handkerchief – and keeping moving are all helpful. The inflammation itself will supply the 'hot', and whatever water is available will provide the cold. Joints can be notoriously painful and once you are able to rest the rule about the waist compress applies; this should also help to take some of the focus away from the damaged joint and afford you some relief.

Just because we have mentioned a reduction in pain as a welcome result of some water-applications, it should not be thought that this is always the primary or safest aim. To stop pain is by no means always synonymous with producing healing. There are situations in which the application of heat can be quite dangerous, as in abdominal inflammations and in acute distress of eye or ear. If some soothing is sought, it may be safely attempted by applying a dry pad, such as a soft woollen scarf. The warmth then builds up from within, and is unlikely to cause distress. Contrast this with a hot-water-bottle applied over an acute abdominal pain: although it might seem like a soothing thing to do it can cause really serious internal injury; just as heat applied to an aching ear may cause rupturing of delicate tissues within.

Where pain is due simply to mechanical stiffness or pressure, the use of alternate hot and cold is a much safer treatment. A tense neck, due to anxiety, will usually relax considerably when hot and cold packs are alternated on its base. Even when the stiffness is due to rheumatoid conditions relief is the usual effect, although it is always possible that a greater pain may result. If this is the case then this indicates that the treatment is unsuitable in this instance and you should discontinue it immediately, for the time being at least.

Water internally

You will have noticed that all the water-treatments we have mentioned so far have been of external application, and this has not been an oversight. We believe that water can be a powerful therapeutic agent when applied to the skin, but if swallowed in quantity or injected into the intestine it is more likely to cause disorder than to improve any natural function. We do not question that the copious water drinking or the use of an enema can make certain symptoms go away or induce bowel movement, but what we do doubt is the wisdom of treating the gut as a drainpipe.

Indeed, it is our observation that drinking an excessive amount of liquid seriously impairs digestive efficiency and the resistance of the bowel wall to toxic substances is seriously reduced when enemas are administered. These topics are covered extensively in the chapters entitled 'Be Kind to Your Kidneys' and 'The Healthy Human Gut'.

On the few occasions when we have sanctioned the use of an enema, a state of panic in the patient is the usual motivation. If an individual is unable to produce a bowel movement for several days, and we cannot persuade him or her that no harm is to be expected because of it, the use of a simple, soapy enema may be less damaging than continued fear. (Not more than one pint of soapy water at blood heat, and retained for about 20 minutes.)

But even so simple a treatment, if it is repeated, can have a negative long-term effect. Apart from aggravating any state of toxic absorption – already referred to – the use of a stimulant to induce what should be a naturally regulated function can be habit-forming. This is quite unlike the effect of cold splashes and cold compresses, which can be used or discontinued freely, and are not habit-forming in any insidious sense – they awaken the skin and vital function in general – whereas enemas give a kind of enervating 'assistance' which makes your bowels progressively more lazy.

Return to normal

You might be one of those individuals who has got used to using enemas as a regular treatment for constipation and who firmly believes that it is impossible for a bowel movement to happen without 'help'. Your 'firm' belief is an appropriate description, and your attitude can only reflect that of your intestines. The principal argument against the regular use of enemas is that they tend to wash away a considerable proportion of material that should be left within the bowel. This is particularly the case with the more elaborate forms of enema, in which large volumes of water are used, or in which rapidly repeated injections and releases of water are produced. If you are one of those people who find such treatments beneficial you would really do far better to cut down your normal food intake by two-thirds, with some Nature Cure guidance about the balance of what is taken, thereby allowing your intestines to make better use of the remaining third.

Drier and healthier

Finally, water-drinking. This is so widely recommended by so many different authorities that you might not believe your ears when we advise strict moderation. Briefly, the troubles so often caused or aggravated by excessive water intake in all its forms, be it plain water, tea, coffee, beer, wine, juice drinks or other soft drinks are these:

1 The digestive juices are diluted, causing delayed and incomplete digestion, with such consequent distresses as dyspepsia and flatulence.
2 The bloodstream is diluted, so that the heart must accept an increased task if the circulation is to be kept at an adequate level.
3 The tissues of the body all tend to absorb a higher-than-normal proportion of water, and this has three effects: (a) The tissues themselves lose tensile strength, so that bruising or tearing occur with relatively minor bumps, grazes and strains. (b) Wastes produced within the tissues tend to remain there in solution, instead of being promptly transferred to the circulatory system for elimination. (c) Some individuals

tend towards water retention and they can become bloated and overweight and this further increases the load on their system as a whole.

4 The kidneys must work harder, to prevent the water-content of the blood rising to dangerous levels. This is doubly serious, because it so often means that the kidneys are less able to carry out their other vital task – the elimination of wastes from the blood. The glib expression 'flush out the kidneys' would be more accurate if altered to 'flush away the kidneys'. And that is neither a cheap joke nor an exaggeration of what can happen to people who habitually drink large quantities of water – however it may be disguised.

5 Excessive drinking leads to excessive perspiration – with undesirable effects described earlier – and this, apart from being uncomfortable, means a corresponding loss of salts from your body.

Summary

In brief, the water cure has a long history, and its main applications have been well tested over the centuries. Special hydropathic equipment may be effective for particular conditions, but generally the true and lasting benefits come from simple techniques that you can perform in your own home. Of these, the compress – in a variety of shapes – is mostly used when feeling unwell. I know some Nature Cure adherents who wouldn't dream of going away on holiday without their 'Wet Pack', in much the same way that the more orthodox thinkers wouldn't go without a packet of painkillers in their washbag.

For everyday use the Squat Splash or shower, the hand rub and cold stamping are the most widely beneficial. Hot and cold alterations are invaluable for strains and sprains, as are the more specialised techniques for emergency use with cuts and burns. Internal use of water should be sparing; large quantities are rarely beneficial, and as a general rule it is more necessary to reduce one's water intake than to increase it.

LIVE WELL. EAT WELL. BE WELL.

Points to remember

1 Water treatments have been used to great effect for centuries.

2 Generally the less violent hydropathic applications are the most effective in the long term.

3 Having your cold splash every morning will soon become a refreshing and invigorating start to the day.

4 Cold waist compresses should warm up within a few minutes and should be removed it they fail to do so. Do not attempt to warm up your compress with a hot water bottle; your body should do the work.

5 If applying a compress or wet bandage to a sensitive area of the body, a waist compress will be needed to balance the effect, and avoid the body using the damaged area as an outlet for excess waste.

6 Quite deep cuts can be successfully treated with simple water and clean cloths. Avoid any antiseptics, keep the area damp and protect with permeable material to allow some air in and gaseous wastes to escape. Don't be afraid to rinse the cut in cold water when changing the bandage.

7 Burns can be successfully treated with cold water. A wet bandage applied and kept damp can be very soothing and aid healing. If using a semi-permanent bandage always use clean linen, not cotton.

8 Do not apply hot compresses to sensitive areas of the body such as the ears or the abdomen, particularly if there is obviously inflammation. Apply a dry soft woollen covering and allow the body to warm the covering and do not use a wet compress.

9 For strains and sprains alternating hot and cold applications can have a better outcome than using ice or only cold packs. Cold compress the injury and balance this with a waist compress at night or when you are able to rest in a warm quiet place.

10 Avoid using enemas even if you feel constipated. Adjustments to your diet and some help with your emotional difficulties or stresses can give you a far better result in the long run.

CHAPTER FIVE

THE FEAR FACTOR

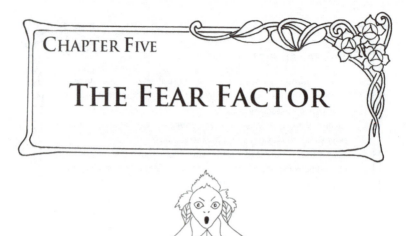

YOU MIGHT WONDER what fear has to do with your health, but fear wears many faces, and the word fear covers a multitude of different actions and reactions. Fear can be a passing emotional state, felt acutely when you see an unrecognised moving shadow in the dark and it can also be a form of unsettling anxiety felt when you have to undertake a task that you have not done before and are unsure of. Whatever form the particular state of fear takes it causes hormones to be mobilised and to circulate around your body. Some are released in limited amounts, and provided that they are accompanied by some physical activity, can actually be beneficial. In other instances hormones can flood your body, as in the case of extreme fear or sudden fright, and this can cause you to respond without thinking, sometimes in ways that are potentially life threatening. Hormones can also be produced in limited amounts but over a prolonged period; this can happen if you are under continual stress at work. This latter situation might seem relatively harmless, but long-term anxiety can cause disruption to normal functioning.

My grandfather was well aware of the significance of fear for a patient and this note in his handwriting was found pinned to the inside of a cupboard:

CONSULTATIONS

Make a routine of asking the patient what he thinks is wrong. The patient's worry is an important part of his condition. You must either set his fears at rest or temper the truth. Persistent fear can preclude any possibility of cure.

Dominant emotions

As one of the dominant human emotions, fear has a far wider range of expression than you might initially suppose. Just look up the word in a thesaurus and you will find that fear has many different names, the commonest may be listed as: fright, distress, apprehension, anxiety, worry, concern, impatience, anger and hate. Some may prefer to call these collectively 'the negative emotions', but it is also valid to regard them as variants or derivatives of fear. Many of these reactions are deep-seated and instinctual and the response may come initially from our limbic system, the ancient part of our brains concerned with survival. Because of this the initial reaction is often completely out of proportion to the stimulus. A horse startled by a flapping plastic bag flees in terror before stopping to look back and assess the real danger. We would do likewise, but we are rarely in the position to be able to flee so we metaphorically move instead, leaping to conclusions about the level of danger involved before taking the time to assess the situation. Of all forms of fear, the momentary grip of fright or the quick wave of anger are probably the least serious. They are closely allied to each other and, in normal circumstances; the system's reaction and recovery take place easily and rapidly. The muscles shaking immediately after helps to dissipate the hormones released into the bloodstream.

Fight, flight or freeze

A healthy release is not possible in many circumstances as we strive to conform to what is accepted and expected from us as normal behaviour. When an animal is startled its sympathetic nervous system is activated. The adrenal glands, which sit on top of the kidneys, flood the body with adrenalin (epinephrine) and the response is usually dynamic and rapid. Depending on its temperament, the animal either flees like the horse, or turns and attacks the trespasser or threat. Either course of action involves intense muscular activity, and a resultant awakening of all vital functioning. The process is assisted by the production and distribution throughout the body of muscle-tensing hormones – the adrenalin flow. This makes possible both more powerful and more rapid actions than in the non-stimulated state. As secondary effects, heart and lungs perform with much increased vigour. For a few minutes, everything is being driven close to the limits, and then, provided the fright or intrusion has not been too serious, the individual may experience the reaction of a distinct feeling of wellbeing. When the immediate danger is over the parasympathetic nervous system is activated and the 'rest and digest' response returns the body to homeostasis. All this, remember, is with creatures inhabiting a reasonably natural environment.

Unfortunately, with our artificial conditioning, we humans are rarely free to respond so instinctively; you are unlikely to show

LIVE WELL. EAT WELL. BE WELL.

physical violence nor are you likely to run away, your conditioning tells you to stay where you are and restrain yourself. But adrenalin floods your bloodstream just the same as it floods an animal's, causing that overall increase in muscular tension with no corresponding vigorous activity to use it up. What might be consumed in a few minutes by wholehearted violent activity instead remains as a powerful influence perhaps for hours. The excessive tension operates worse than uselessly, it makes you feel unhappy and the continued muscular tone consumes energy without producing any compensating activity. Although the parasympathetic nervous system will attempt to balance the excess of hormones, without the vigorous activity associated with fight or flight to use them up it takes a long time to return to normal levels.

That is bad enough, but worse follows. If the situation goes on for any length of time then vicious cycles begin to develop involving vital function and mental ability. For example, prolonged tension in the muscles of the neck may affect the nerves that control digestive activity; the resultant indigestion gives rise to emotional irritability, which in turn may set up further strain in the neck muscles.

Animals

As we now know due to the mapping of the genome we are closer to apes than we are to the big cats. Both apes and cats can be startled, but their responses are strikingly different; whether wild tiger or domestic pet, the cat instantly turns to face the intruder, ready to strike back. The primate's immediate initial response is to run for safety, then to turn and see what it was that frightened them. They may ultimately decide that attack is the best course of action or they might just keep a safe distance. We should not be ashamed, then, of our natural tendency to be afraid; it is probably one of our most powerful strategies for survival. Although us humans are expert hunters, deprived of our weapons we can quickly become the hunted.

We are not unique in our ability to think of the future, there are other animals capable of forethought, but we do project our fears into it probably more than other animals. The anticipation of conditions such as pain, unhappiness, hunger or shame can be intense. Most of us quickly forget what real pain felt like, but recalling an embarrassing situation can be as distressing as the actual event. It seems reasonable that our fears for the future are also most intensely concerned with situations involving other people, and the possibility for loss of self-esteem.

Professor Steve Peters[1] describes the immediate primitive response that comes from our ancient limbic system, as our 'Chimp'. Our limbic system responds on an emotional level, instantly and instinctively, without any pause for consideration about the situation. He describes in his book *The Chimp Paradox* how we need to nurture and manage our Chimp using our logical frontal cortex, the 'Human' part of our brain. In this way we can learn to understand and manage the way we react in frightening or stressful situations.

Simple, unreasoning fear can drive any of us into actions that given just a second of rational thought would obviously be illogical and even potentially self-destructive. For example, you are driving a car on a busy road, and are so distracted by the relatively trivial incident of a yellow and black striped insect landing on you that you overreact in fear, and risk losing control of your vehicle. A normal sensible conscious intelligence can be completely gripped

---

1 Peters, Professor Steve, *The Chimp Paradox*, Vermillion Books, 2012.

by fear, and it is then that we do stupid and illogical things. When we are in this state, various bodily responses become apparent. One of the most obvious is your mouth going dry.

Pale and parched

From the above examples, it should be easy to see the deeper and more lasting significance of fear. We experience worry, or deep anxiety, as a prolonged version of fear, and our nervous system and guts can be seriously affected by these negative emotions. Just as your mouth becomes parched, a similar thing happens with the lining of your alimentary tract as it ceases to produce its natural secretions. In the same way as you go pale with fright or white with anger, the blood vessels of the stomach wall become constricted. If you are in a state of agitation, or are worried about something you will not be able to digest food properly; the digestive juices, starting with those in saliva, can be more or less completely absent. If you do eat when you are emotionally distressed you will often experience the feeling of 'the food going down in lumps'. It is neither properly masticated nor is it exposed to the first stages of digestion in the mouth. Many of us in this state of worry or anger will often try to stuff the emotions back down our throats with food.

Stomach ulcers

Less immediately obvious is what may happen to your stomach as a result of extended worry. The pale, bloodless lining lacks its essential oxygen supply, and deprived of normal nutrition and waste-removal processes, becomes devitalised. This is in some ways not unlike the predicament of frostbitten fingertips, in which a proportion of the cells do not recover when circulation is eventually restored. However, whereas a mild frostbite merely results in painful irritation, a devitalised stomach lining is a different matter altogether. The enzymes in the stomach are designed to break down protein, and the moribund cells of the lining are just that. If enough cells are in a nearly dead state, the corrosive juices break through the surface. Unlike the surface cells, which are capable of withstanding stomach acid when they are in their normal, healthy state, the tissues behind the surface have little resistance when assaulted by peptic juices. This is the beginning of a situation in which degenerative changes may continue, ultimately leading to serious ulceration. More recent research has found that the bacteria Helicobactor Pylori is the cause of stomach ulcers, but as they are around us, and inside us at all times the above information still holds good; they can only take hold when the conditions are suitable for them to multiply.

Contacts

If we explore the comparison between the effects of cold and of fear, one could say that brief fright, like a brief application of cold water, may be quite beneficial. It is good for your mind and body to come into contact with life's realities, and if these occasionally happen to be uncomfortable they are often no less valuable for that.

With modest shocks, the initial effect is usually unwelcome and unpleasant, but provided you have the reserves available to respond and react healthily, *and are not prevented from being physically active*, you should subsequently have a much longer period of euphoria. We have all experienced this in everyday near-accidents. The more frightful the catastrophe might have been, the more severe the immediate shock. There is the sudden grip of fear and the slow, horrid sinking of the stomach, then the gradually developing counter-effect of relaxation and raised spirits.

Tensions

So why is sustained tension so serious? In most parts of the body, blood vessels have to share their space with muscles, and often when the muscles are in contraction – that is, in the fattened state – the veins get compressed. When the muscles are normally active, alternating between tension and relaxation, the intermittent pressure upon the blood vessels can be entirely beneficial. There is a positive assistance to the circulation of the blood and the lymphatic system relies heavily on the adjacent muscle actions for efficient circulation. Sustained muscular tension, however, has no such helpful effect; it is fundamentally obstructive.

This is most easily felt in the strong muscles in your neck. If you press the muscles when your neck is tense it is like touching the back of your hand; there is no give. With a healthily relaxed neck, the feeling will be more like that of the heel of your hand, with a thick pad of soft, pliable muscle. So it follows that when your neck muscles are tight, the veins may be almost completely flattened, this prevents the full escape of deoxygenated blood from your head, and makes the arrival of fresh blood almost impossible.

All physical and vital function, as well as mental activity, depends on adequate circulation, so the detrimental effect of sustained constriction requires no explanation. It should also be stressed that the nerves also suffer as much as any other tissue when deprived of adequate circulation; starved nerves may become inflamed and so directly produce still further tension, and related pain in the muscles under their control.

Tone

All muscles in a normally healthy state have what is called tone. This means that they are slightly active even when resting. There is a modest tension, which ensures both a rapid response when action is required and a precise obeying of the control messages. There is also a modest production of warmth, which helps to keep the muscle soft and flexible. Because all muscles in a state of healthy tone are similarly involved they do not produce obvious movement – the limbs, for example, remain at rest, because all the tensions balance out.

Where tone is lower than normal, the individual is usually relatively unfit. Poor tone means slower responses when action is called for, often with a lack of precision and a lowered efficiency. Any saving of energy that might result from the too-relaxed resting state is heavily outweighed by the wastefulness when in action. Although not directly related to states of fear, poor tone may be one feature of severe shock, the exhaustion of nervous energy that can result from any of the negative emotions, if it is intense or prolonged enough.

More frequently, it is excessive tone that is associated with acute fear. The person is described as being 'highly strung' or 'hyper-sensitive'. This implies too great a production of muscular force even when apparently at rest, unfortunately this state is usually associated with a too-rapid or exaggerated response when move-ment is attempted. It may be difficult to accept, but a person sitting quite still in this over-stressed state may be using up more energy than another, calmer person moving around quite actively. Their vital organs will be driven unfairly hard, and therefore it is not surprising if, at the end of a tense but relatively inactive day, they are quite exhausted.

Balancing act

To clarify the negative effect of serious stress, here are some examples of the physiological situation. Fundamentally our muscles work in pairs, so for each prime mover or agonist muscle there is an antagonist muscle that has a governing and balancing action. This activity not only controls the way that the prime mover acts; it also contributes to muscle tone. Tone is maintained by the constant and passive partial contraction of our muscles. When these muscles are working harder than they need to due to extra tension, then more energy is used than in normal daily functioning.

Whatever your reserves, excessive muscular tone dissipates them at a disheartening rate. When negative emotions are at work and producing a lasting condition of internal conflict – of one muscle working against another, of pressure obstructing blood-flow and of nerve-function being disorganised – your available energy is being burned up wastefully. There is no positive activity associated with it.

Impatience

Impatience is a situation in which the incidence of fear may not be immediately apparent. It can accompany pride, ambition and material success, and so suggest confidence and greater-than-average ability. Yet somewhere, deep down, there will be a streak of self-dissatisfaction. The suspicion of inadequacy may never be consciously sensed, the impatience being directly induced by the body's unconscious intelligence. Yet, all that you may be aware of is a small, gnawing doubt about the ability to carry your plans through to completion.

Anger and hatred

Next time someone makes you angry, try to take a little time afterwards to think about just what it was that disturbed you. The likely reason is fear in one of its many guises. It may have been the fear of being physically or emotionally hurt by the other person's thoughtlessness or selfishness. Or it could be fear of becoming involved in a potentially embarrassing situation – one in which your normal feelings of self restraint have been challenged by deep, instinctive pressures.

Feelings of fear and hate can so easily be roused by what we see as the misdemeanours of others. But these purely negative emotions are of no positive use to us and are more likely to cause us harm than have any beneficial effect on the situation. True humanitarianism must have a positive, active and constructive content and potential outcome. In much the same way it doesn't do you any good to be ashamed, apologetic or repentant, unless these moods ultimately lead to constructive action.

Purpose

Simple fear has a purpose, just as pain has a purpose, and to have fear of pain may be a perfectly healthy response. If your fears have grown too big, or are with you too much of the time, you must seek help to understand what is magnifying them. But it might help to realise that we tend to be more fearful when we are run down. A lack of sleep makes us more tired, our confidence is reduced and our thinking can become muddled. Our responses become slow and our energy reserves get run down. Both consciously and unconsciously we recognise that we are not in a condition to deal with problems or even routine tasks effectively. We can therefore easily become worried about our difficulties, be startled by trivial incidents and lose patience with ourselves when things do not go right. We tend to have a feeling of general foreboding, to be unreasonably afraid of the dark, or of heights, and to imagine that people are noticing our failings – all of which may be far more imaginary than real.

There is nothing to be ashamed of in experiencing fear, and it may be more intensely felt if you are a healthy and intelligent person than it would be by someone who is ailing and/or behaving irresponsibly. To tackle your debilitating fears we must first try to identify them, and then attempt the often long and painful process of working back to their origins. If this is possible, the effort is well spent. Some fears have causes that are deeply buried in your unconscious; however you should be wary of too much self-critical self-analysis. An objective and perceptive outsider may be able to make helpful deductions. Some of the talking therapies can be helpful and Cognitive Behavioural Therapy can assist us to see that our reactions to situations that may have been apt at one time in our lives, are no longer applicable, helpful or appropriate.

Posture

The posture you adopt if you are a fearful person has a direct effect on your confidence. To allow your head to drop forward, over a collapsed chest and with your shoulders raised up around your ears and with your core muscles loose, might feel like you are protecting yourself and avoiding being seen in the world, but such a posture aggravates many of the physical causes of fearfulness. Tense neck, cramped chest and unsupported digestive organs all contribute to mental and physical inadequacy and poor functioning.

To try to assume an attitude of self-confidence can allow and encourage improvement in many of your vital processes, and eventually enable you to develop true confidence. If there is one activity that can help you to deal with the physical aspects of fear it is walking. This provides activity for your whole system. It removes you from the oppressive environment and it gives you an opportunity to have some mental and emotional space.

Keeping moving and active is really beneficial and sometimes walking is not possible, so the next best option is deep rhythmical breathing. Even if the air is less fresh than you would like, vigorous respiration brings at least four benefits to the nervous or anxious person: The movement helps to release tensions; opening up the chest improves the posture and assists circulation; the nerve cells enjoy better oxygenation; the rhythm of breathing can have a steadying effect on your nervous system. Try breathing in for a count of seven and out for eleven. This can have a steadying effect and you can do it anywhere. Breathe through your nose and allow your body to relax.

A sense of proportion

One young male patient who, many years ago, was a member of a discussion group at the Kingston Clinic, was talking about his gloomy fears and anxieties and how he dealt with them, and said, 'I keep them written on cards in a cupboard and each week I take them all out and lay them on the table. I look at them, one by one, and then put them carefully back in the cupboard until the following week. When I bring them out again, most of them have shrunk a little; some are no longer relevant'. It is an interesting idea perhaps, and in his case it was tempered with a reasoning mind. This simple exercise means that you can recognise, but do not have to become obsessed with, your fears; instead engaging in a deliberate exercise to keep them in proportion makes it possible to ultimately dispose of them.

A few notes on Mindfulness

There are many books on the market dealing with Mindfulness, usually in the form of self-help publications. It is certainly in tune with Nature Cure thinking — to be present, aware and learning to slow down and take stock, which are very useful life tools.

But it is only human nature to grasp at whatever the health industry is hailing as the next 'great white hope', especially if you hope it can solve all your problems painlessly. However, this is rarely the case and the practice of Mindfulness will only stick and be truly helpful if you can incorporate it easily into your overall healthy life strategy.

If you can learn to be at peace with yourself and find some calm in an increasingly busy world it can only help you to maintain your mental, emotional and physical health. But don't forget, you will still need to work at all other areas to have a balanced healthy life — eat well, live well and be well.

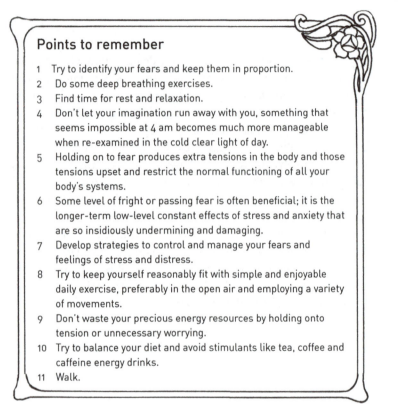

Points to remember

1 Try to identify your fears and keep them in proportion.
2 Do some deep breathing exercises.
3 Find time for rest and relaxation.
4 Don't let your imagination run away with you, something that seems impossible at 4 am becomes much more manageable when re-examined in the cold clear light of day.
5 Holding on to fear produces extra tensions in the body and those tensions upset and restrict the normal functioning of all your body's systems.
6 Some level of fright or passing fear is often beneficial; it is the longer-term low-level constant effects of stress and anxiety that are so insidiously undermining and damaging.
7 Develop strategies to control and manage your fears and feelings of stress and distress.
8 Try to keep yourself reasonably fit with simple and enjoyable daily exercise, preferably in the open air and employing a variety of movements.
9 Don't waste your precious energy resources by holding onto tension or unnecessary worrying.
10 Try to balance your diet and avoid stimulants like tea, coffee and caffeine energy drinks.
11 Walk.

LIVE WELL. EAT WELL. BE WELL.

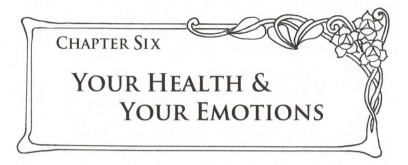

CHAPTER SIX

YOUR HEALTH & YOUR EMOTIONS

AN AGE-OLD teaching of the Nature Cure school is that you cannot be well physically if you are emotionally disturbed. The psychologically troubled individual who is unhappy, worried, fearful, resentful or in a distressed state of mind will almost inevitably find these emotions being expressed through a sick body. Equally, if you are in a state of continuing physical discomfort or pain, depression can easily set in.

Nature Cure places the same level of importance on mental as physical health and always has. When my grandmother wrote her first version of this thesis there was no information from any orthodox source on the subject of mental health. Rather than accept that mental ill health was a normal, albeit pathological, aspect of being a human, the authorities shut people suffering from mental illness away in institutions. These patients were often treated harshly with electric shocks and confinement. I remember patients staying at the Kingston Clinic who were suffering from what would now be called Post Traumatic Stress Disorder and our approach was to treat the whole person, not only their mental distress. Fortunately, nowadays the orthodox approach is rather more enlightened and there is an emphasis on talking therapies such as Cognitive Behavioural Therapy. As such these therapies are non-invasive and broadly acceptable to the Nature Cure way.

Counselling in its widest sense is a major part of any Nature Cure consultation; you talk, we listen. Then we look at how your mental distresses are affecting your overall health. Assuming that your material and everyday basic needs are being met, two of the most vital necessities for good health are emotional balance and a positive mental outlook. What many people still find difficult to understand is the idea that you might have become ill because you are in such a state of emotional turmoil that your body cannot function normally.

Fear

As we have explored in detail in the chapter entitled 'The Fear Factor' a great deal of confusion and upset can be brought on by fear in all its guises and this fear affects every part of your body. We usually think that our brains register danger first and send messages via the nerves to initiate a response. Groundbreaking work by Research Professor Candace Pert[1] has shown the response is often too rapid for this to be the case and in fact every cell of our bodies responds instantaneously to a perceived threat. So far from the brain taking in the initial stimulus and sending a signal to the guts via the vagus nerve before the guts respond, your head and viscera act together. This brings about a feeling we are all familiar with – the gut reaction. This is the case with an instant fright response, and in the past we would have used up the adrenaline that was released with a rapid and life-saving flight. Sadly the things that are likely to instil fear these days are unlikely to make you take flight, you are more likely to freeze, and this means that often the reactively released hormones circulate in your body causing you discomfort for several hours. Passing emotions can be widely disturbing to all your bodily systems, but a lasting state of anxiety must take a large share of the responsibility for the undermining of our psychosomatic balance.

Let us suppose that you have experienced a pain, maybe in your stomach, or it could be in your chest, and that it has persisted for a few days; long enough for you to imagine disturbing pictures of something thoroughly unhealthy and unpleasant. You begin to worry that it might be the first symptoms of something really serious. Seeking consolation, you look up the symptoms in a book or, more likely the Internet, and find all manner of alarming illustrations and disturbing text; your worst fears are confirmed. Your anxiety levels rise, nervous tensions increase and your blood pressure rises and this affects your circulation. The initial pain has now risen to a barely manageable level and you feel distinctly unwell. In this anxious and frightened state you consult your doctor, fully expecting to be given a diagnosis and told the worst.

As a rule Nature Cure practitioners prefer not to give conditions specific names, we believe that to do so can give the nature of your complaint too great a significance, and therefore too much power to inspire fear. Going to your doctor for a diagnosis might appear to be a sensible step if only to get a name for your problem, even if you ultimately have little faith in the medicine that will be prescribed. But the alternative approach can be so much less distressing, that is, trying to understand what your body is telling you. Most discomforts and disorders are in fact indicative of an effort by your body to heal itself, cleanse its tissues and eliminate accumulated wastes. The concept is fully explained in the chapter 'The Healing Crisis'. Looking at illness like this can immediately create a more confident and co-operative attitude. The pain that had been so frightening becomes more bearable and the nervous and muscular tensions that aggravated it have relaxed.

Despondency vs confidence

Your friends and relatives can play a major role in how you perceive your illness; they have the potential to push you along the road to dejection and despair, inadvertently feeding your fears. They might have known somebody who had the same condition as you who had to be 'so careful for the rest of their lives', and although their concern is real and any comments they make are with the best of intention, they can still make you feel hopeless. Alternatively they can lend you a sympathetic ear and a shoulder to cry on, but also encourage you to see the possibility of complete recovery; the more confident you can feel about your future the greater the potential for a full recovery.

Try to be positive

Being ill is not much fun and can dishearten you overall, but seeking a goal in your life that you want so much that is worth overcoming your illness to achieve, can be a real impetus to start down a more positive road. It is crucial to believe that *it is possible* to be the assured, healthy person you would like to be. Try to picture yourself not only as healthy, but also as *doing* the thousand and one things that you can do only if you are healthy. Chose one and do it. Every journey of a thousand miles starts with one step. As my grandfather so often reminded his patients and his associates, 'Health for health's sake is neither so urgent nor so inspiring as *health in order to do something.*'

Look beyond

Even when an unfortunate diagnosis has been given and confirmed, this is no reason to accept defeat. Recognise that the situation is serious, give it your wholehearted attention, but don't become hopeless. The life force is on your side, and there can be no more powerful ally. Even if the condition confronting you has 'always been in the family' do not let it take over your life and destroy you, try to see beyond it. The incredible innate powers of intelligence and regeneration within your living body are beyond human comprehension. Live for each day as fully and as optimistically as you can. Fear can cast long shadows, step out of those shadows and start to believe in your body and your future.

It can be too easy to blame someone or something else for your ill health. It is true that there are some for whom this is correct if, for instance, you come from an abusive family you will inevitably be starting from a point of disadvantage. But, if you are reading this chapter, then you have already found the strength to take steps to help yourself.

You might have been fortunate enough to have had a good start in life, but now you are ill. Rather than accept that your life choices have led to your current state, you seek to blame Providence. However, this state of affairs has considerably more to do with cause and effect and we believe it is the purpose of the Life Force that we should be healthy and that we should live life to the full.

Arnold Bennett[2] expressed the potential:

It is rather fine, this tense bracing of the will before anything worth doing can be done – I rather like it myself – I feel it is the chief thing that differentiates me from the cat by the fire.

Nutrition

It is quite possible to completely undo the beneficial effects of good, honest, balanced, natural feeding by being over-anxious about your diet. No matter how good the advice you may have been given, or how carefully you try to follow it, you are always in a state of some anxiety in case you should make a mistake over this food or that, concerned that you might have taken a little too much of one or not quite enough of the other. It is not what you do occasionally that does the harm; it is the unhelpful daily habits that have a cumulative effect on your health. We are only human and it is normal to fail in our ideals sometimes. If you have too much cake, too much coffee or too much alcohol on a single occasion, let it pass without self-reproach. Don't beat yourself up about it. What's done is done; just try to engage a little more self-control in the future. This will get easier as your body gets healthier and the desire for healthy foods will dominate.

Analysing every mouthful, worrying over it, and later checking any passing symptom is both weakening and self-destructive and as an added downside, it can make you quite difficult to live with. Worse still, this kind of worrying about your basic nourishment can effectively poison even the most wholesome food and drink. 'Mental dyspepsia' inevitably expresses itself in muscular tensions, which leads to physical indigestion and consequent malnutrition.

Our belief is that sanity in diet can possibly be best summed up in this simple guide: Get your food as right as you can, enjoy what you eat *and then forget it*!

Mealtimes

Mealtimes should be happy and relaxed. Unfortunately, it doesn't matter if you eat in splendid isolation or with your family or friends, they can too often be used as an opportunity to mull over or bring up domestic problems, resulting in a stressful situation. The court jester of mediaeval times, whose duty it was to keep the diners' minds off serious things, helped many stomachs to cope with otherwise appalling and indigestible meals.

When we worry, or are angry about something, the tension that results can cause blood vessels to constrict and at mealtimes the flow of digestive juices is also inhibited. Destructive emotions don't only sour our vital tissues and fluids, but they pervade our mental attitude as well. On the other hand, there is nothing to equal a relaxed happy frame of mind for an efficient flow of digestive juices and an enjoyable situation.

It is the orthodox approach to think of the mind as the organising manager of our physical body, but as we have already noted the two work simultaneously so the regular action of the heart and lungs, digestive activities, protective reactions and a thousand and one other complex functions are psychosomatic. Mind/Body. In other words; they involve your mind and your body concurrently. Some processes may appear to be almost unaffected by your mind's condition, while others are immediately and obviously changed by it. Good health requires equilibrium – and equilibrium is good for your health.

Smile

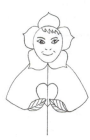

Believe it or not, if you can make yourself smile at the people that you meet it creates a positive feedback to your brain. The movement of the facial muscles prompts your brain towards a more positive outlook. As already discussed, talking about your physical disorders with friends can sometimes magnify them rather than reduce them, however much apparent enjoyment there is in talking in interminable detail about the most miserable of our symptoms.

If you are feeling down, it is all too easy to become obsessed with the destructive activities of mankind and feel pessimistic about the future. Whether it is climate change, wars, laws, government decisions, the decline in the global bee population, human over-population or any of a myriad of conditions affecting the planet, we can find much to cause us stress and distress. It would be foolish, of course, to disregard all that is mad and anti-life, but you should try to avoid dwelling continually on the appalling possibilities. Rather try to find positive actions that you can realistically take.

We believe that our thoughts and our emotions determine and create the atmosphere around us, and that everyone who comes within it is affected by it in one way or another. So even if you are not particularly concerned about your own health, you might still contribute something positive to the wellbeing of those with whom you come in contact. With this in mind you would do well to take some responsibility for your own mental attitude. Try to act as if you are not down or depressed, and if you can keep doing this you can often eventually help yourself out of the negative habit.

Strive to forgive your enemies; obviously, at certain times and in certain circumstances real forgiveness is impossible, but for everyday disagreements don't let bad feelings fester and grow, they do nothing for your wellbeing. You could even try to project friendly thoughts toward them; this can be as much an act of self-preservation as the putting up your arm to ward off a physical blow.

Insecurities

In her work with children, my grandmother estimated that emotional insecurity, in its many facets, was a major disruptive factor in more than half of the many physical ills of childhood.

No one can measure the suffering of an envious child: there is no age too young for envy to arise and cause damage and the emotive injury may take some considerable time and a huge amount of understanding from the parents to repair. We are not talking here of normal sibling rivalry but of a pathological spiteful attitude. The emotional insecurity can arise from emotional starvation, and this can be one of the most seriously distressing situations of childhood.

Talking therapy

At any age, if you are emotionally disturbed you often simply need an opportunity to talk it out, not so much sharing as shedding your burden of guilt, whether real or imagined, or expressing your feelings of self-dissatisfaction. All you want is a listener who will not be shocked or express any disapproval, and in speaking out about what troubles you, often a solution starts to formulate itself. Until you experience this release your striving for health can be severely handicapped. You might be one of the relatively few individuals who, when presented with an explanation of the physical and emotional causes of your illness, are capable and strong enough to take on the task single-handed. But for the majority of us it is almost impossible to carry out and interpret an honest self-analysis. Usually, we make far too much out of a trivial error or weakness while carefully overlooking the major defect.

Another long-established belief in Nature Cure circles is that you cannot enjoy true and lasting health unless there is harmony in the three major aspects of existence, the physical, the mental and the emotional including the spiritual aspects. This holistic concept helps to explain why it can be so frustrating to attempt one form of treatment after another if you are stuck in an unsatisfactory relationship or in a job that makes you really unhappy. Dissatisfaction or frustration with those closest to you, or your occupation, can make the rebuilding or maintenance of good health quite impossible.

Skin troubles may be frequently associated with such a situation, and the place of the family background in your distresses should not be overlooked. There are families in which skin disorder and breathing difficulties – eczema and asthma – are closely interlinked. Both symptoms are usually related to a long-established catarrhal background, but the physical factors are only part of the story: most often we find serious emotional stresses. The agonising struggle of an asthmatic attack, like the intolerable misery of the eczematous skin, seem to be the outward signs of the deep, hidden and sealed in emotional upset. Nor is it a matter of simple excess stress, the characteristic feature is conflict: not merely the unfairness of a heavy burden but the doubt about how to cope with it, or even whether it ought to have to be coped with.

As a rule, when the patient is a young person the parents are not the best people to handle the situation. Often they constitute a major part of the stressful and conflicting background. We also regularly see that it is a parent's own unresolved emotional tangles that are transferred to, and expressed through, the unfortunate child.

Growing up

This above situation does not mean that when you grow out of childhood you are entitled to continue to throw the blame for all your unhappinesses on your parents. Every person you meet, all your friends and all your enemies, and every experience you have undergone have played a part in building up your personality. This ought to enable you to be more understanding of your parents'

LIVE WELL. EAT WELL. BE WELL.

problems, and so gradually allow you to cease to regard them as the antagonists in a perpetual conflict. We all fail to achieve perfection in our relationships to a greater or lesser extent, and perhaps we should regard the situation as a challenge, even if it is sometimes a daunting one. The satisfaction will be so much greater when we have managed to achieve a happier conclusion.

If, for any reason, your marital relationship has broken down and you now live apart, there is particular need for self-control in the presence of your child or children. No bitterness or recrimination should be indulged in, and although your feelings of loyalty may be severely strained they must not be broken. Whatever awkward questions your child asks you, your answers must be simple and straightforward, with no hint of complaint or of self-pity, otherwise the child will feel it their duty to offer comfort and protection to you. This would be entirely unacceptable, and would almost inevitably cause your child deep unhappiness and tensions leading ultimately to a state of ill health. This ill health might not present in a physical form but can cause the child to withdraw and they can become silent and uncommunicative. In this situation professional help should be sought.

Middle age and the menopause

Far from childhood, there are the emotional difficulties of middle age and onward, more often characterised by depression than by any excess of excitement. Perhaps women are the greater sufferers, because of the double setbacks of the fundamental changes in their family relationships and the internal adjustment of the menopause. Whereas the man may find his work becoming increasingly burdensome, the woman may find her whole life losing its accustomed patterns.

As we tend to live longer, and maintain a better level of physical fitness into an older age than our parents, many of us take up activities and pastimes that are often challenging and made possible only because we now have that bit of spare time. Lesley Kenton[3] in her book *Passage to Power* illustrates that the menopause can be a great opportunity for positive change in a woman's life, far from being the end it is the start of a new phase. And it is certainly not a foregone conclusion that it needs to be medicated, nor is it something to be afraid of, it is a natural change from being a fertile woman into a freedom from monthly periods and any fear of unwanted pregnancy.

Of course this can be a sad time too, as your role is changing, but it is a completely normal process and if you have been reasonably careful with your health there is no reason that it should be any more of an upheaval, or distressing, than the menarche. Worrying unnecessarily over what might happen at 'the change' can make you ill, and this can bring you down and rob you of your ability to cope. Instead look ahead positively to your third age. Welcome the time you have to yourself, especially as, more often than not, the children will have left home. It is quite normal to feel sad that your brood has grown up and flown the nest – empty nest syndrome is very common – but these days they have a bit of a habit of appearing back on the doorstep every now and again wanting to stay at home between jobs or relationships. There may be adjustments to be made particularly if your husband or partner has retired at the same time. You might be blissfully happy with the company and do lots of things together, but it can also be a period in which you take stock and have a good hard look at your other half and decide that now might just be the time for a complete life change.

To stay in a marriage or relationship that is no longer serving either partner well can have devastating effects on your health, and on the quality of your lives. Indeed, middle age is a time for some deep contemplation and review.

Quiet contemplation should of course be part of your everyday life as you get older whichever sex you are. Quiet for meditation; quiet for healing of mind and body; quiet for restoring and maintaining your sense of values. It should not be a time for self-torturing introspection and the churning over of regrets for what might have been. There is no point in going back over things that cannot be undone, middle age is time to say, 'that was that. Now what?'. Trying to look forward with a mature eye can help to lift feelings of depression, it can help to change your mood for the better and this can allow your circulation to improve, your headaches disappear and your personal outlook take on a better perspective. By quiet solitude we don't necessarily mean hiding away in a darkened room, sometimes that might be just what you need but generally we recommend quite the opposite. Most healthy people find it is infinitely more effective if their quiet time takes the form of a walk, in the country for preference, but failing this, anywhere that the air is clear and cool. Breathe deeply, walk with purpose, listen to the birdsong and enjoy the views. Ralph Waldo Trine[4] wrote, 'subtle and powerful are the influences of the mind in the building and rebuilding of the body' and this certainly does not only apply to your younger years.

Work

Many people like to believe that overwork is a great factor in bringing on premature old age. Yet some of the busiest people we know are the happiest and certainly they look the youngest. It is the conflicts and indecisions that are so often associated with non-creative or uncongenial work that are the truly destructive features. Endless hours at the computer or working on piles of paperwork can wear you down faster than honest muscular exertion.

So how long should we expect to live and be active? It should not be how long, but how fully, that really matters. For those of us who have a zest for life, it is excellent to evict from our minds the old chestnut of threescore and ten. At 74, Verdi produced Othello, at 80, Falstaff. At 80, Goethe completed Faust. At 85, Titian painted his memorable picture Battle of Lepanto. So, for most of us, there is still plenty of time!

Peace

Glowing, vigorous health is worth any effort that the human mind and spirit are capable of, but it is something that only you can achieve and maintain for yourself. By all means seek help and advice and find friends who can share in the exercises and activities that help to keep you young in outlook and attitude, but your personal approach to your life, and your state of mind will determine your new way of life. No other person can do this for you, though they might be able to help you along the way. Until your heart is freed of fear and negative emotions, until all thoughts of revenge are discarded and until any desire for power is rejected, there can be no lasting peace on earth or honest well-being in any person.

References

1   Candace B Pert. *Molecules of Emotion*. 1997.
2   Enoch Arnold Bennett. Journalist and author (1867–1931).
3   Lesley Kenton. Passage to Power. 1996.
4   Ralph Waldo Trine. Philosopher, teacher and author. (1866–1958).

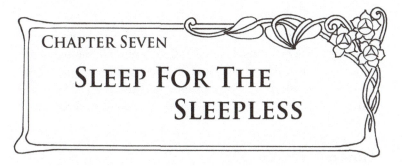

CHAPTER SEVEN

SLEEP FOR THE SLEEPLESS

GETTING ENOUGH sleep is a basic requirement for us all to be able to function normally. It is really important that you don't skimp on it. If you don't get enough sleep and rest, your body soon starts to let you know. All sorts of metabolic activities, as well as essential repair and rebuilding work, go on while you are asleep. Deprive your body of sleep too often and these activities will be compromised.

Sleep is amazing if only for the effect it has on your body. Small cuts miraculously heal overnight, stubbed toes recover and tired muscles are revived. Sleep allows the problems that loomed large and insurmountable the evening before to be put back into perspective before the morning. Also, it is now known just how important sleep, rest and recuperation are for the healthy functioning of our brains. Recently research has shown that although the brain is not served by the lymphatic system that generally transports wastes from around the body to the cleansing organs while we are asleep, it does have a glymphatic system. The team carrying out the work in the University of Rochester Medical Centre[1] has found that this glymphatic system bathes the brain cells and washes out toxic wastes. But, it can only do this while we are asleep. So if you lose out on sleep, your brain loses out on these vital cleansing efforts.

This team of neuroscientists also identified that the brain only has limited energy at its disposal and if there is not enough sleep time the brain will have to choose between vital functions; awake and aware or asleep and doing the internal housework. This could partially explain the fuzzy thinking of the individual deprived of sleep.

How much is enough?

Many different research projects have investigated the negative effects of lack of good quality sleep, and they broadly agree that most adults need between 7.5 and 9 hours sleep every 24 hours. Irritability, weight gain, heart disease and a lack of ability to concentrate can all have their roots in lack of sleep. Lower productivity, the inability to remember and consolidate information and increased incidences of depression are also connected to insomnia. On the other side of the coin, research has also identified that it is possible to get too much sleep. Adults who are taking more than 9 hours sleep every night are likely to be low on vitality and at an increased risk of illness and accident.

The amount of sleep you need will vary with age and the differences between the needs of a new-born baby and an elderly sedentary subject can be vast. It really does not matter which chart you consult, all are in broad agreement about the hours of sleep needed for each different age group. In adulthood, 8 hours per night is considered normal. However, some do appear to need less sleep than others, these are people who can apparently burn the candle at both ends. There are likely to be genetic reasons for this, quite apart from the differences in lifestyle and other day-to-day factors.

The best conditions for sleep

To get the best possible night's sleep you need to establish some basic routines. Regular broken nights, even if you spend the full 8 hours in bed, can still result in a sleep debt. Many people, including quite young children, have televisions or computers in their bedroom and some high-achievers even work right up to turning out the lights and getting ready for sleep. Bedrooms are often stuffy, with windows kept shut, or only open on warm summer nights and the central heating on until late in the evening. Those who eat their evening meal later in the evening often find difficulty getting a good night's rest. These late meals are usually heavily starch and protein based and often accompanied by an alcoholic drink or a cup of coffee. With all these factors at work it is no wonder that sleep time is fitful, punctuated with periods of wakefulness, worry, and vivid dreams which stop sleep being as restful and rejuvenating as it should be.

Chronic sleep loss

The Great British Sleep Survey (2012)[2] also found that in the UK sleep difficulties affect up to 80 per cent of people over 60 years of age, while 67 per cent of total respondents reported bodily discomfort as the reason for poor sleep. 34 per cent identified their partner's sleeping habits as the major disturbance. 36 per cent identified the reason for their poor sleep as their environment, and this included room temperature, external noise and light levels. The survey went on to identify the thoughts that were most likely to keep you sleepless as, 82 per cent, what happened today and what needs to be done tomorrow, 79 per cent, how long you have been lying awake, 76 per cent, trivial thoughts and 71 per cent fears about the future and worrying about the past.

Getting your full quota of sleep is important for many reasons, but it doesn't necessarily need to be all in one chunk. Considered physiologically, it appears not to matter so much when the sleep is obtained so long as the total, week by week, is sufficient to meet your body's requirements or an average of 56 hours.

Some popular misconceptions about insomnia

Ask any nurse who has been on night duty in a large ward and they can always tell stories of heavy snorers who, night-after-night, keep all the other patients awake. Their idiosyncrasy is almost always the same; when told by other patients of their snoring they quite sincerely protest, 'But I didn't sleep a wink all night'. As they see it, the snoring must have been the work of somebody else.

So, if when you wake up in the morning and you just know that you 'didn't sleep a wink all night' you might be surprised, and perhaps a little relieved, to learn that you are generally mistaken. We do not, ordinarily, know when we are asleep; the essential outward symptom of sleep is that we have lost consciousness. We sleep but we do not remember the fact, therefore you cannot be sure if you did or did not sleep. Only someone who deliberately stays awake for hour after hour through sheer willpower can be certain that they did not sleep a wink. My grandfather believed that the gathering of this precise knowledge was not worth the effort or the misery.

It is common for people to go off to sleep and then wake up in the middle of the night and start to fret about their problems, and then not be able to get back to sleep again. In *The Chimp Paradox*[3] Professor Steve Peters explains that when we are in this sleep/wake state it is our 'chimp', or our emotional brain, that does the thinking. His makes the useful suggestion that you gently put your chimp back to sleep, then tackle the problem with your refreshed logical brain in the morning.

To understand why insomniacs believe that they are sleepless, we must remember that sleep is essentially rhythmic. It comes in waves throughout any normal sleep period. The larger phase of this regularity has a direct connection with the day/night circadian rhythms. Most of us sleep better at night although this is not a universal habit throughout the animal world. Most humans choose to sleep at night when it is dark, even if there is wide variation in the times we spend in bed. Some turn in early and get up with the lark, and others rarely go to bed before midnight with a later start in the morning. The latter group are more likely to build up a sleep debt if they also have to get up early for work but cannot believe that they will be able to sleep before midnight.

For even the soundest sleepers, the depth of sleep is not constant. The healthy child or muscularly active adult in good health may appear to sleep the whole night through, without once breaking through into consciousness. But at frequent intervals throughout the night, for a few seconds at a time, they reach a stage just short of wakefulness. Even when we are most soundly asleep, awareness is never very far away, for instance if you tickle the nose of someone soundly asleep with a feather, they will bring a hand up to brush away the hypothetical fly without the slightest interruption of any of the outward indications of sleep, and generally without any later memory of the event.

Beware the drug habit

It is a common misconception that unconsciousness and sleep are one and the same thing. From this misunderstanding arises the widespread acceptance that certain drugs and sleeping pills can produce genuine sleep. It is all too easy to become hooked, and to believe that sleep is impossible without them, but in truth, genuinely restorative sleep is almost impossible in a drugged state. It might seem like a good idea to just take a little sleeping pill, especially when you are quite convinced that you have been lying awake night after night and you feel that your life is becoming impossible.

There is a variety of sleeping pills that are currently being prescribed; these include anti-histamines, selective GABA medicines, sleep-wake cycle modifiers, benzodiazepines and tricyclic anti-depressants. Each one comes with its own list of side effects. Quite apart from clinical experience, good old common sense tells us that these solutions to your sleeplessness are best avoided. Too often it was observed at Kingston Clinic that in reality there was nothing fundamentally wrong with the patient's ability to sleep, until it was artificially affected by the medication.

More than ten million sleeping pills are given each year in England alone.[4] So it is a widespread problem and one that most of us will experience at different times in our lives. According to sleep specialist Professor Kevin Morgan[5] of Loughborough University's Sleep Research Centre 'sleeping tablets treat the symptoms of insomnia, not its causes'. He goes on to say that 'non-drug treatments have been under-used, but they offer the best long-term solutions to chronic insomnia.' His team have been researching the benefits of psychological treatments including behavioural change and self-help to promote better sleeping patterns. In addition, The Great British Sleep Survey (2012)[4] identified that those taking sleeping pills were 85 per cent more likely to feel helpless, 74 per cent more likely to feel alone and 49 per cent more likely to feel their sleep was out of control than those who were not taking sleeping pills. So, natural approaches are the safest, best and longest lasting remedies for sleeplessness.

If you are unable to sleep well at night it is worth trying to make up for the shortfall with catnaps or 'power' naps during the day. Sometimes just a few minutes can be enough to enable you to function much more efficiently. Many people find it impossible to sleep for short periods during the day without feeling awful, but this would indicate a sleep 'debt' and a real need to work on night-time routines. It can take a bit of training to get yourself into the habit of taking a short snooze when you really need to catch up on lost sleep, but it is well worth it and certainly nothing to be ashamed of. Night shift workers often find that a short nap during a break time can help them prevent accidents and poor decisions. Whichever way you accumulate the hours of natural sleep you need, getting enough is vital to your health.

Sleep blessed sleep

So how can you help yourself to have a better, more refreshing sleep? You might need to change longstanding habits that have

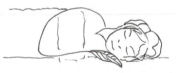

been contributing to your problem, and that can be very hard to do, but it is often essential. In their useful book *The Sleep Solution*, Nigel Ball and Nick Hough[6] give a 21-day programme to better sleep. It is all common sense, solution based information and their recommendations are delivered in the form of a step-by-step guide. There is not enough room in this book to do more than make the following, hopefully helpful suggestions:

Twenty suggestions

1   Have a reasonably firm mattress that will support your body well, but will also encourage you to turn over regularly during the night. By changing your sleeping position during the night you assist your circulation and give different parts of the body some rest from the pressure.

2   Don't sleep on your back. This can make the work of your kidneys harder and makes you more likely to snore.

3   Don't use more covers than you really need.

4   Have a window or two open for fresh air. Your body should be warm and under the covers but your head should be cool and there should be plenty of fresh air. However, avoid sleeping in a draught.

5   Don't have heating on in your bedroom while you are sleeping. Unless the outside temperature is in the double figures minus Celsius, your covers should be sufficient to keep you warm. If it's really cold use a hot water bottle rather than an electric blanket.

6   Try to go to bed around the same time each night. Create a simple bedtime routine that works for you.

7   Avoid coffee, tea and caffeinated soft drinks (cola drinks, Irn Bru, Red Bull etc), for at least six hours before going to bed. Yes, we all know folk who can drink coffee or Coke last thing at night and still sleep 'well', but caffeine is a stimulant and just what you *don't* need before preparing to sleep. This also includes alcoholic drinks that have caffeine in them.

8   Don't eat a heavy meal within three to four hours of going to sleep. Sleeping on an empty stomach will almost always

give you a better night's sleep despite the commonplace habit of the 'wee something before bed'.

9 Try to avoid indulging in heavy physical activities – be it bricklaying or dancing – within two hours of bedtime.

10 Don't watch TV or stream anything on your laptop or tablet immediately before going to bed. Leave the work e-mails until the morning, when you will be thinking more clearly anyway.

11 Don't have a TV or computer in your bedroom. Your bedroom is for sleeping, and for sex too, but primarily it is for sleeping and getting your much needed rest.

12 Try to put your worries on the back burner and don't try to resolve problems at 4am. Your worried 'Chimp' will magnify them, they will look much more manageable when you use your logical brain in the morning anyway.

13 If your children, partner or pets wake you don't get upset about it; after you have dealt with the problem go back to bed and let the problem go, don't get agitated about the loss of sleep.

14 Don't get agitated if sleep is eluding you. Do some deep breathing and try to relax.

15 If you are struggling to get back to sleep after waking in the middle of the night, try applying a cold waist compress. With the usual proviso of warm-up time (See the chapter 'Water and Nature Cure' for instructions). This will help you to relax and sleep will be more refreshing.

16 Try 'pretending' to be asleep. Curl up in your usual sleeping position and breathe steadily as if you were asleep. If wakefulness persists, stretch your arms above your head; take a deep breath and change your position.

17 Try the Buddhist breathing technique of clearing your head of all thoughts and just concentrate on your breathing. Don't change the way you are breathing, just observe it. If thoughts come back, clear them and return to the rhythm of your breathing.

18 Try counting backwards from 9,999. It helps to stop the thoughts that are troubling you taking centre stage.

19 Try going through the different parts of your body and relaxing each in turn, starting with either the toes or your head whichever works best for you.

20 Try not to get up in the night and start making cups of tea, you will only need to get up again to go to the toilet.

These suggestions can be hard to follow through, but it is worth persevering and finding the ones that work for you. A technique that works in one situation might need to be adjusted for another. Keep trying and remember to relax!

References

1 The journal Science, 15 August 2012. The work of neuroscientists Dr Nedergaard at the University of Rochester Medical Centre.
2 The Great British Sleep Survey (2012).
3 Peters, Professor Steve. *The Chimp Paradox* 2014.
4 The NHS website 2015.
5 Professor Kevin Morgan of Loughborough University's Sleep Research Centre.
6 Ball, Nigel and Hough, Nick *The Sleep Solution* Vermillion Books 1998.

PART TWO

The following eight chapters cover the conditions most often seen at the Kingston Clinic, and in our outpatient practices. There are also the topics most often talked about at the regular Round Table discussions and Friday Question Time at the Clinic. The simplest treatments most effectively applied are also described.

The original works, many of which are still available as monographs, came out of the periodical "Rude Health" that James Thomson and Leslie Thomson published between 1947 and 1979. Their words of wisdom are still pertinent and serve to underline how well the Nature Cure principles have stood the test of time.

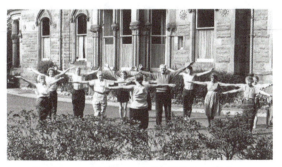

Exercises on the lawn at the Kingston Clinic

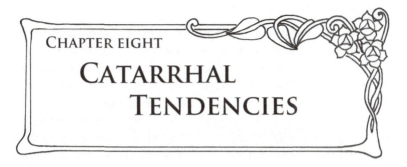

CHAPTER EIGHT

CATARRHAL TENDENCIES

WE ALL KNOW WHAT it feels like to have an acute catarrhal condition like a cold or flu, stuffed up and a little hot in the head. Noses run, throats feel sore and glands are swollen. We tend to think of catarrh as only affecting our noses and throats but it is condition that can affect any of the mucous membranes that line various internal linings of our bodies. This includes our gastro-intestinal tract and any surfaces that need mucus to absorb, assimilate or protect. The thickened mucus that comes out as discoloured phlegm is carrying waste materials for removal by the simplest and shortest route.

This condition in one form or another, is so widespread that it is possibly the most important of all simple diseases, and the way that you treat it and deal with it will decisively influence your future health. Rationally handled with a Nature Cure of 'intelligent leaving alone', a catarrhal system is capable of rectifying itself in an almost astonishingly complete way. But in more advanced cases you might suffer from tonsillitis, sinusitis, or earache.

When things are in an abnormal state and there is overloading of your blood-cleansing organs – the skin, the kidneys, the lungs and the liver – it is comparatively easy for your body to use the mucous membranes for supplementary support. When this happens the mucus becomes much thicker, more profuse and usually discoloured. The membranes themselves become swollen and painful, so that for instance swallowing is painful and breathing through the nose is difficult. The simplest way to treat this is to take no food for a day or two and liquid intake should only be sufficient to meet real thirst – these steps will lessen the load on your vital organs. Your body's energies are freed up to concentrate on the immediately important job of eliminating the excess of acidic wastes. If you are unable to take time off work to allow your body the space it needs to do the work, then a simple fruit fast for a few days with as much rest and relaxation as you can take, might have to suffice.

Natural guidance

The symptoms themselves often give us a clear indication of the actions we need to take. One of the commonest aspects of a head cold is the loss of taste, but it's not your tongue that has become insensitive, your tongue can still identify the four basic tastes: salt, sweet, sour and bitter – but the linings of your nose which have become so thickened that the sense of smell is dulled. Without smell, most food flavours are lost and food can become unappetising. If you add to this is positive discomfort in swallowing, the logical step is to give meals a miss until the acute stage is over.

Deliberate disregard

Nature is generous with her warnings when you are not living as healthily as you might, and poor lifestyle choices are very often to blame for illness. It might be only human nature but most of us have trained ourselves to ignore warning signs and the fitter you are to begin with, the more likely you are to push on regardless, and to brush aside impatiently the indications of lifestyle error.

If you suffer from too-frequent colds, or have an almost continual excess of secretion from any mucous membrane, then you would be wise to take this as a sign that something is fundamentally wrong. If you take the analogy of a safety valve for a common cold then when there is excessive activity of the mucous membranes there is the potential for a waste of vital energies.

So what is the cause of catarrh?

It would not be unreasonable in the majority of cases, in Britain at least, to lay the blame for excessive mucus on overconsumption of starchy and sugary foods. Overeating of almost any kind can produce a similar effect, but the processed and refined carbohydrates so often found in junk foods are often the most troublesome. However it is also possible to overeat cooked proteins or fats, particularly now that palm oil has found its way into so many manufactured foods. What connects these foodstuffs is that they all have a poor complement of vitamins and organised minerals, relative to their energy-producing potential.

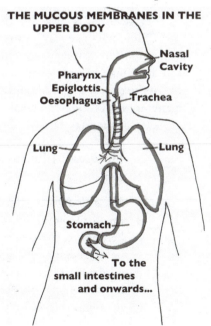

THE MUCOUS MEMBRANES IN THE UPPER BODY

Nasal Cavity

Pharynx

Epiglottis

Oesophagus

Trachea

Lung

Lung

Stomach

To the small intestines and onwards...

This means that there is a greater creation of acidic wastes and this results in a slow but progressive accumulation of residues. These accumulations throw strains onto the blood-cleansing organs and they become less efficient as a result. To break this vicious circle, an elimination process is initiated and active catarrh is the result.

An unbalanced diet is not the only cause of a catarrhal state. Lack of adequate fresh oxygen circulating can result in excessive waste build up even if your diet is fairly good. Poor occupational posture can add further strains on your vital organs, so that their full function is compromised. Added to that, a general lack of muscular exertion hinders the circulation of the blood and our largest organ, the skin, has only limited participation.

Your stomach is probably the most immediately distressed organ, although there may be no obvious symptoms. The stomach is an astonishingly tough and resilient organ, but we tend to drive it to the brink of breakdown on a regular basis. In this state, it is kept more or less inflamed, and this makes it easy for the lining membranes to become catarrhal. Catarrh then interferes with the efficient functioning of gastric digestion.

How will I know if I have a catarrhal condition?

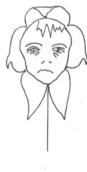

My grandfather stated that, 'those who over eat of bread and grain foods are invariably constipated' and he went on to explain that such constipation may not be immediately recognised, because it can be present even when there is a daily movement of the bowels. So if you regularly over-eat starchy foods there are one or two signs to look for: your tongue may be large, heavily

LIVE WELL. EAT WELL. BE WELL.

coated and showing tooth marks (indicating that the tongue is too bulky to fit comfortably within the lower jaw.) Flatulence may be persistent. Your bloodstream is likely to be overloaded with the products of combustion – incompletely neutralised because of a lack of organised minerals, and inadequately eliminated by your overworked kidneys. In the mornings you might wake up feeling sluggish.

However, if you are also actively catarrhal, there may be no immediate danger. Your vital organs are saved from serious breakdown by the elimination of acidic excess through the mucous membranes. But don't be tempted to try, or accept, some form of treatment that could be successful in stopping that catarrhal activity. To take one simple instance, nasal catarrh is distinctly troublesome: it causes a feeling of stuffiness, difficulty in breathing, loss of sense of smell and the annoyance of your nose running constantly. There are several substances which can be inhaled to cause a shriveling of those swollen mucous linings. It seems almost miraculous that within quite a short time you can breathe freely and forget your tissues.

But, unless at the same time you are prepared to make radical changes to your normal routine of eating and drinking, your body must do one of two things: either find some alternative route for ejecting the wastes or store them within your body. When a simple and superficial flow of mucus is obstructed, the alternative must be a storing of the wastes in a deeper, and usually more vital, structure. Denied escape through the nose, the catarrhal material may try the throat or the ear. To employ an analogy, the body organises the process, and it is not too misleading to imagine the somatic activity putting a squeeze on the unwanted material. This like toothpaste in a tube, which has pressure applied and erupts through any hole in the container; if there is no hole open, and the force is great enough, the weakest spot in the wall will rupture. In the human body the result may be a septic sore throat, or an inflammation of the middle ear. These are the acute manifestations, and they are certainly drastic and uncomfortable enough to command your immediate respect and attention.

Infertility

There is perhaps no predicament so demoralising as the discovery that you cannot conceive when you long to have children. Most of the specialists who deal with this problem can provide extensive information about timetables and techniques, but they tend to overlook the fundamental question, 'why should it be difficult?'

Psychologists may talk understandingly about the emotional difficulties but the physical factors can easily be overlooked even though they are probably predominant in the situation. It is perhaps putting it rather too starkly, but often when there is sterility it indicates that conditions are unfavourable for the production of healthy offspring. Of course, there are many considerations that, in individual cases, make nonsense of that claim, but it nonetheless seems to be in line with nature's preference for giving the next generation the best chance of success. However, we do not think that apparently infertile individuals should accept defeat and become despondent nor do we think that heading for IVF or other invasive techniques is a good idea. We would prefer that they accept the challenges and do something really positive about improving their collective fitness and systemic health to a level consistent with the importance of parenthood. The start they can give their child will be so much better for it.

Good for both

There is no need to apportion blame or even to determine which partner is responsible for the failure. It should never be forgotten that one feature sets true Nature Cure apart from every other form of treatment, 'Nothing which we do or suggest for a sick person could harm a healthy one.'

That may seem like an inconsequential claim, but it has enormous significance. It cannot weaken you to follow a healthy, balanced diet and a lifestyle that includes deep breathing and outdoor exercise, even if it has been designed to revitalise your partner. There is no question of adopting unnatural methods, which are more likely to interfere with your long term health, than to assist a normal conception and a successful pregnancy.

The long view

In very many cases, it is not unusual to find that either you or your partner is a typical catarrhal subject. Your secretions can be so abnormal in content and so laden with acid wastes that the normal chemistry and physics of conception are completely obstructed. To correct the situation may take some months, maybe even a few years. But most couples will agree that it is much more sensible to provide the best possible physical background for new life, rather than adopt short-term shock tactics with all the attendant anxieties and the potential for a less-than-perfectly healthy child. Most potential parents are in the younger adult group, although this is changing with the desire for a career before settling down to have children, so, the number of years that have to be compensated for by your new living habits will vary depending on your age.

To bring your secretions back to a normal composition, all the things which are good for clearing nasal catarrh, watery skin, sluggish kidneys, inactive lungs, waxy ears, gassy stomachs, 'froggy' throats and sticky eyelashes are just as useful and important. Anything you can do that helps to clear acid excess from one part of the body relieves some of the strain from every other part. For infertility it is good to eat lots of green leafy vegetables not only because of the traces of vitamin E – the 'fertility vitamin' – that they contain, but because of their useful complement of the organised minerals that do so much to neutralise the excess wastes you are carrying around in your body. Sterile, processed, salty, sugary, over-cooked food is not the stuff upon which to build human fertility. All food should be as fresh and living as possible, and as wholesome and organic as circumstances allow. Fresh air breathed deeply helps to burn up acid wastes in your blood and tissues, converting them to carbon dioxide which can be breathed out, this means that they will not be clogging up your vital function.

Making those necessary changes

There is no point in beating about the bush – there are no shortcuts; when your body has been obliged to concentrate wastes within its own tissues, the task ahead is considerable. With your full understanding and co-operation, and Nature Cure assistance in the form of external, non-invasive treatment, the time taken to mobilise and eliminate the wastes must be proportional to the time during which the disease condition has built up. There is a rule of thumb that says that you should allow a month of treatment for every year that your condition has taken to develop. It is a useful rule of thumb, but it is by no means mathematically accurate. So much depends upon your perception of 'the disease'. Sometimes pains which have plagued you for several years are eased almost completely within a few days; in other cases, a joint which has been immobilised for only a short time may take many months to revert to something like normal function. That is, the particular symptom which is most annoying to your intellect may be well down on the body's somatic list of priorities; long before a uric acid deposit can be uplifted from your painful toe joint, your kidneys must be revitalised and your entire bloodstream brought back to more or less normal chemical constitution and balance.

It is human nature to want to give things names, and the catarrhal condition certainly attracts more than its fair share. To quote just a few: head cold, blepharitis, rhinitis, tonsillitis, hay fever, sinusitis, stomatitis, otorrhoea, mastoiditis, goitre, bronchitis, asthma, gastritis, mastitis, gallstones, kidney stone, colitis, cystitis, vaginal discharge, fibroids, eczema and oedema, are all but different names for various facets of the same basic condition.

Louis Kuhne, two centuries ago said, 'Just as there is but one health, so there is but one disease; tissue uncleanliness.'

Today we do not accept this to be a complete explanation because there are always factors other than the purely chemico-physical that are significant, yet fundamentally his observation is true. To avoid any or all of the conditions listed above, it is necessary only to ensure that your body does not hoard its wastes.

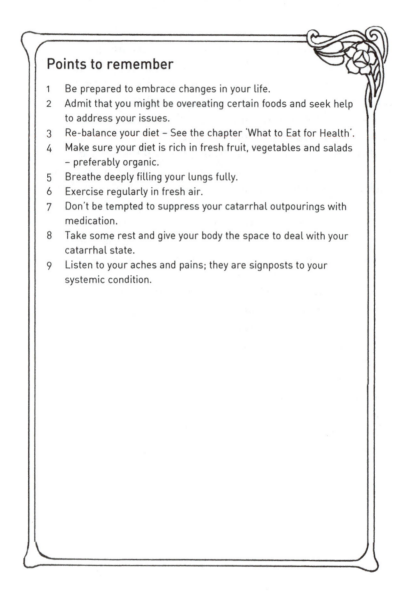

Points to remember

1   Be prepared to embrace changes in your life.
2   Admit that you might be overeating certain foods and seek help
    to address your issues.
3   Re-balance your diet – See the chapter 'What to Eat for Health'.
4   Make sure your diet is rich in fresh fruit, vegetables and salads
    – preferably organic.
5   Breathe deeply filling your lungs fully.
6   Exercise regularly in fresh air.
7   Don't be tempted to suppress your catarrhal outpourings with
    medication.
8   Take some rest and give your body the space to deal with your
    catarrhal state.
9   Listen to your aches and pains; they are signposts to your
    systemic condition.

LIVE WELL. EAT WELL. BE WELL.

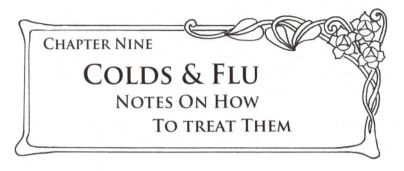

CHAPTER NINE

COLDS & FLU
NOTES ON HOW
TO TREAT THEM

No more antibiotics

In the waiting room at a recent visit to my dentist I noticed that there was a pile of leaflets issued by The Scottish Medicines Consortium entitled, 'Get well soon without antibiotics'. It is widely recognised that colds, sore throats and most coughs are 'caused' by viruses and mostly these are self-limiting conditions. Antibiotics simply don't work on viruses, yet the medical profession have happily been prescribing them for years to patients who mistakenly believed that the pills would make them better. Until now, when the crunch has come and over-use of antibiotics has rendered them useless in many cases. Now the word is that these colds, sore throats and most coughs will simply get better on their own. So how can that be when we have always been told that the body needed to be 'helped'?

No Mystery

As we have already explored colds and acute conditions are healing processes and we accept that there are viruses that can 'cause' colds and flu, and they are all around us and easy to be in contact with. So the question is, 'how come not everyone gets the malady that is doing the rounds?'

For any virus to take hold and start to proliferate there needs to be a pre-existing condition and the tissues need to be in a receptive state. In the case of colds or flu the latter condition is what the older Nature Cure practitioners would have called tissue uncleanliness. Many people develop a cold soon after getting chilled in bad weather, but you should ask a few questions. For instance, would it not be fair to say that the person was unusually sensitive to cold at that time? Had they been made particularly miserable for the level of dampness or draught? Was it more a feeling of general misery than of genuinely reduced body temperature? Was there a true chilling of a vital organ such as the liver or the kidneys? Was it of a significant degree and duration? In most cases it would be justifiable to say that the feelings of chill and the development of a cold are only different aspects, or successive stages, of a healing crisis.

Crisis

A typical cold goes through several stages, and at any given moment different kinds of internal cleansing and adjustment may be in progress. Thus, after the first outward elimination takes place, there may be a brief feeling of relief as the blood flows more freely. But within an hour or two, perhaps far less, the partly cleared blood picks up even greater amounts of waste from the tissues. The patient now feels much worse; the next stage has been reached. Breathing may be obstructed by excessive catarrhal flows; the mucous membranes become tender and stingy; the brain is fatigued and incapable of normal levels of function; the patient feels chilly, runny-eyed, short-tempered, resigned, weak and feeling very sorry for themselves and a nasty cough is starting to develop.

These are the outward indications of a remarkable cleansing

and rejuvenating process within, and above all there is a need to recognise that the body is fully occupied with its own self-improvement.

Influenza

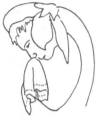

Influenza is essentially 'a cold writ large', and has very similar causative roots. People who live in such a way as to acquire many colds are also prone to develop flu. But much depends upon how you treat your cold. With an increasing awareness of how you can live more healthily, each successfully conducted cold should minimise the need for flu. But that is a generalisation and a simplification, you may have to contend with so many adverse factors in your daily life that a couple of colds each year and a bout of flu every second or third year may be inevitable. But here again it is important to be quite clear that influenza, in itself, is no cause for panic. Properly understood, and handled with calm, confident intelligence, it is a constructive process. The fear with which so many laymen and doctors regard flu is due to the violent potential of the condition when it is mishandled. A good going flu involves a greater width and depth of reparative and eliminative activity than a common cold. The body as a whole is more completely committed to the task, and there are greater deviations from normal balances than in a cold – eg there is real fever, and the nervous system is often deeply disturbed.

Whereas with a cold the principal effect on the mental state is of depression, with flu there is usually greater distress. For one thing, the fever is usually accompanied by some degree of disorientation by day, and unpleasant dreams by night. Actual delirium may occur at some stage in more severe case. With a cold, lack of interest in food is common, in flu there is more likely to be a vigorous upset in the gastric function. The bowels may also participate, so that exhausting vomiting and diarrhoea add to the patient's misery. Headache may be more than just a dull nag; there may be severe neuritic pains extending down the neck and into the shoulders. The mucus inflammation is liable to be severe, and any cough can be a real punishment. Teeth, bones and muscles may all add their own characteristic pains to the general misery. Perhaps worst, for many people, is the combined feeling of uselessness and unavoidable panic about the flu 'going on forever'.

A typical attack of flu may last from anything between a few days and two or three weeks. Often it takes place in two distinct stages, with a false 'recovery' between. This is when if you are an impatient patient you can so easily set yourself back; you think that you are feeling better and being under pressure from work or family commitments you are tempted to try to resume normal life and activity too soon. Persuading yourself that the attack is over you plunge into an attempt to catch up with your personal backlog, only to find to your dismay that your body was really only pausing briefly before pressing on with the second instalment of intense activity.

'Killer Flu'

Stressing the point, because it is of vital importance, the severity and after-effects of any cold or flu are dependent upon how it is treated.

A few paragraphs from my grandfather's report on the Great Flu Epidemic may underline the message:

During the Epidemic of 1918 over 150,000 deaths were
registered in Great Britain, and this by no means completes

the statement. Many hundreds of thousands of patients were left with serious heart symptoms, lung trouble, deafness, visual disabilities, anemia, catarrh, insomnia and other enervating ailments. My own personal experience, along with that of many other Nature Cure physicians, with whom I have discussed the matter, is that Influenza is neither difficult nor dangerous to treat, nor are debilitating symptoms an inevitable outcome.

Reports collected from Naturopaths practising in all parts of the world after the 1918 wave—the most serious in living memory—gave a death-rate of under two per cent; whilst around them in the same cities, among the same types of people and under almost identical conditions except for the treatment, the death rate was from seven to over 30 per cent. In my own practice, during the epidemic of 1918, I had personal charge of 87 cases. In 86 of these cases my instructions were faithfully carried out, and in no case was there either death, complication or any lingering sequel. The majority of these patients spent two or three days in bed, felt somewhat shaky in their walking for a further day or two, and within a week or two actually felt better than they had done before the attack. In the one remaining case my instructions were wilfully ignored, and I was forced to discontinue.

He went on to emphasise the need for the successful Nature Cure adherent to grasp firmly the Naturopathic understanding of acute disease. This has already been explained in this chapter, but just to re-emphasise the point here is a further quotation from his work on Influenza:

Hippocrates recognised acute disease as having a constructive basis, and in his teachings constant reference is made to eruptions, colds and fevers, as being the outward evidence of the body's vigorous effort to cleanse itself. This is exactly the teaching of the Nature Cure School today. The eternal verities do not change.

Types of flu

There are four main types of flu and, no matter how novel the identifying names given by epidemiologists and immunologists, any particular case consists either of one of the following types, or of a combination of two or more:

1 RESPIRATORY: This starts off with violent, paroxysmal coughing, and is most likely with the extremes of youth and age. Suppressive treatment can easily result in lasting respiratory disturbance.

2 GASTRO-INTESTINAL ('gastric'): Nausea, vomiting and abdominal pain are the immediate indications, often progressing to diarrhoea. Suppressive treatment may lead to chronic digestive or liver disorders.

3 NERVOUS: Headache of unusual severity, accompanied by pains in neck, chest and upper abdomen. Depression and sleeplessness are common accompaniments. Erroneous treatment may lead to congestion in the brain and inflammation of its coverings, or other forms of nervous disorders.

4 FEBRILE: Quite intense fever, sometimes accompanied by disorientation, to the extent of delirium. In this form, it is imperative that no nourishment whatever should be given to the patient until the fever has subsided. It is probably in this type that it is most easy to prejudice the patient's recovery by well-meant 'kindness'. Offering tempting

delicacies, or providing sweetened drinks might seem to be innocuous but can seriously undermine the work that the body is undertaking. Suppressive treatment may lead to a wide variety of consequences: eyesight, muscular strength, the heart, kidneys, skin, lungs may all suffer.

Reassurance

The foregoing list is intended mainly to reassure the Nature Cure adherent that even quite violent symptoms, provided you stay calm and do not become fearful, are no cause for alarm. There is no need to attempt a differential diagnosis before applying sensible and helpful treatment. No matter which organ or tissue is most obviously or severely under stress, the general approach is the same for all types.

As soon as the condition makes itself evident, you, the patient, should resign yourself to a few days in bed, with nothing whatever to eat and even limiting fluid intake to sips of plain water. Usually, you will be restless and your neck muscles will feel hard and tense. Simple gentle massage to these may give considerable relief; alternatively, providing you are used to them, a compress on neck and waist should be applied with some success. Such compresses may be renewed every 1½ to 2 hours, always ensuring that they warm up promptly and remain so. For fuller information about compresses see the chapter 'Water and Nature Cure'.

If your headache is severe and persistent, it may be permissible to apply mild symptomatic treatment by placing a hot-water bottle at your feet. This action tends to draw away any excess of blood from the head by 'derivative effect', and should not be regarded as anything more than a temporary relief. In extreme cases, you might feel lethargic to the point of being comatose, and a compress broader than the usual waist type may be justified. Suggesting that the compress be enlarged to the size of a small towel but always made of thin cotton or linen material, and that the woollen covering is a blanket rather than a scarf is not too drastic. If you are very feverish there should be no difficulty in obtaining a good, warm reaction. Note, however, that no attempt should be made to bring down your temperature with prolonged cold bathing or the application of ice packs. These activities can seriously interfere with your body's reparative processes.

Progress

Once the initial acute misery has passed (usually in 48 to 72 hours), and the temperature is more or less normal, light nourishment may be offered. Naturally sweet fresh fruit, such as ripe apples, pears, grapes and the like are best. It is essential that these are organic and free from pesticide residues. If no organic fruit is available avoid imported grapes and stick with locally produced fruit. Small quantities of fresh green salad are equally suitable, again this should be organic out of preference. Fluids should be taken only in tiny sips, and be neither chilled nor hot nor sweetened. Sugary drinks such as the proprietary glucose preparations are to be avoided completely. Diluted syrups of real fruits, such as blackcurrant or rose-hip, should be treated with caution. They consist largely of refined sugar and have an undesirable content of preservative sulphur acids.

By this time, the need for frequently changed compresses should have passed, and perhaps three in any 24 hours will suit best, morning, afternoon and night time. Beware of feelings of euphoria at the passing of the initial misery. You can easily get the false impression of being 'just about well again' and attempt some strenuous physical or mental activity. In this state getting seriously

LIVE WELL. EAT WELL. BE WELL.

chilled or over-tired is all too easy. On the bright side it is possible that, if you can control your impulses and keep resting, you will make a steady recovery, and be more or less fit in another two or three days! More likely, in any but the lightest flu, it will become obvious that a second phase has to be faced. Usually far less acutely physically distressing than the first bout, but it may make up in duration what it lacks in intensity. Feelings of frustration, uselessness and general depression are common. At this stage also, the unpleasant features may be greatly reduced by avoiding more than a bare minimum of food and drink, and avoiding physical or emotional stress.

Points to remember

A simple recommended procedure in handling a typical bout of influenza:

1 No food whatsoever for the first 48 to 72 hours, not even the most innocent-seeming fluids such as fruit juice or milk.

2 Quiet and rest in bed until the fever and shakiness have cleared. No visitors; No decisions; Forget the outside world.

3 Consider applying compresses to waist and neck, but first be sure you know exactly how to apply them.

4 Avoid all stimulants, whether in the form of drink, food or drug. So-called 'health' drinks, whether taken hot or cold, are often seriously disturbing because of some unsuspected ingredient, and 'natural' restoratives often contain alcohol or caffeine.

5 Do not let pride stand in the way of returning immediately to bed if sitting up proves unexpectedly tiring. Avoid any risk of chill.

6 Remember at all times that influenza is an intelligent effort by the body to throw off accumulations of waste and to restore more normal balances within.

7 There is no danger in influenza provided the foregoing points are observed from the beginning, and no attempt is made to stop what the body is trying to do.

8 Fear is more deadly than fever, and understanding what is happening to you removes fear. See the chapter 'The Fear Factor'.

9 Trust your body's somatic intelligence.

LIVE WELL. EAT WELL. BE WELL.

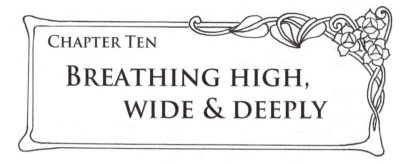

CHAPTER TEN

BREATHING HIGH, WIDE & DEEPLY

IN THE PRECEDING chapters we have looked at catarrh, cold and flu and one of the first signs of these conditions is that your breathing is affected. We all need adequate supplies of oxygen to enable our bodies to produce energy but for it to be really effective we have to be purposefully involved. To enable the body to take in enough oxygen we have to have some way of exposing a large area of delicate tissues to the air, and a means of transporting the oxygen to all other parts of our bodies. The surfaces of the lungs have to be easily permeable by gases; this absorptive tissue is thin walled and therefore must be protected from external injury. This is why it is always protected with a thin layer of mucus, and it is this protective mucus that thickens to an abnormal level when we have a catarrhal state.

Why is deep breathing important?

Bringing oxygen into the body is the primary function of the lungs but no less important, although secondary in sequence, is the expulsion of wastes. Blood returning to the lungs carries waste products and these are mainly acidic and include carbon dioxide. These gaseous wastes are removed from the lungs with each exhalation.

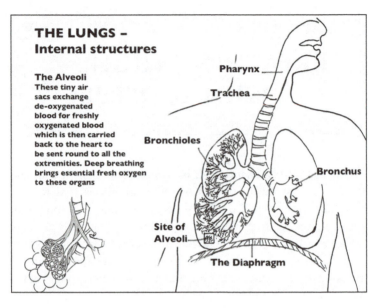

THE LUNGS –
Internal structures

The Alveoli
These tiny air
sacs exchange
de-oxygenated
blood for freshly
oxygenated blood
which is then carried
back to the heart to
be sent round to all the
extremities. Deep breathing
brings essential fresh oxygen
to these organs

Pharynx

Trachea

Bronchioles

Bronchus

**Site of
Alveoli**

The Diaphragm

For the majority of us, work entails sitting or standing in a fixed posture, often with our spines curved and the rest of our bodies virtually motionless except for some small activity of hands and fingers. This would be an impossible situation if it weren't for our automatic mechanisms of breathing. This means that even when our body is at rest, the thorax is unconsciously working. The chemical processes and the functioning of all of our vital organs are heavily dependent on a good supply of oxygen, as is the nervous system, including the brain.

Because of our almost universal adoption of the curved posture, be it over desk, bench, table or sink, breathing occurs automatically principally by the action of the diaphragm. But when we exert ourselves our chest begins to heave, and with this really full breathing takes place. The heart responds instantly to inhalation getting ready for the newly oxygenated blood coming through and increases its beat rate, falling back as we exhale. You can check this for yourself; just put your fingers on your pulse at your wrist and note the beat at rest, now take in a deep breath and the rate will rise slightly and fall again as you exhale.

If you are a reasonably healthy person and have become too engrossed in something whilst sitting still for a long period of time, your diaphragm will have been carrying out the basic minimum of respiration, but every now and then your unconscious controls will attempt to stimulate costal breathing; your ribs heave and you will sigh. When the diaphragm alone is in control of the breathing, the effect is to draw the lungs downward and at the same time your abdomen protrudes. By contrast, when the ribs are mainly involved, the lungs are expanded forward and upward, with usually some flattening of the abdomen. The latter occurs because as the ribs open out they draw up the sides of the diaphragm and at the same time widen it.

Ideally, both diaphragm and ribs should each carry out their fair share of the work of respiration. The fullest inhalation is produced when the ribs are raised as the diaphragm is pulled down. Either movement alone may produce an expansion of the thorax but the real potential is realised only when the two work in unison. Anything that obstructs the free movement of either must reduce the efficiency of your breathing.

Range

Equally important to vigorous breathing is complete exhalation – the bulging upward of the diaphragm and the falling inward of the ribs. It is the difference between the fully expanded and the fully contracted capacity of the chest and represents the individual's

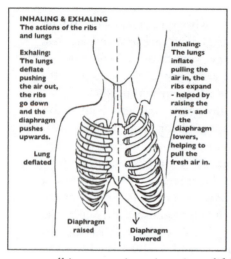

INHALING & EXHALING
The actions of the ribs and lungs

Exhaling:
The lungs deflate pushing the air out, the ribs go down and the diaphragm pushes upwards.

Lung deflated

Inhaling:
The lungs inflate pulling the air in, the ribs expand - helped by raising the arms - and the diaphragm lowers, helping to pull the fresh air in.

Diaphragm raised

Diaphragm lowered

'swept volume', or the bulk of air shifted with each full breath. This is usually only during the most intense exertions. All of your bodily functions demand oxygen and produce waste gases, and the automatic controls of respiration usually maintain a tolerable level of supply. However, in the absence of vigorous activity, this is far from generous. When you are deprived of the stimuli of walking, running, jumping, lifting, dragging, laughing and shouting, your breathing is maintained at a low level. This means that there is precious little reserve of oxygen in your tissues, and a state of near-starvation can gradually develop.

Wasting

Without realising it, you begin to slow down; your thinking and your actions become slower and can lack precision. Health has many levels, and too many people are resigned to living lives barely free from discomfort, for them, the 'occasional sigh' is probably a lifesaver. Without it, the upper regions of the lungs can remain quite immobile, and the ribcage becomes similarly inflexible in its upper segments. When your lungs become immobile, in the same way as any other inactivated part of your body, they tend to lose their full functional ability. Added to this, if your health is poor it is liable to become a dumping area for your body's

LIVE WELL. EAT WELL. BE WELL.

excess of wastes. Should these wastes reach a sufficiently high concentration the lung tissues may suffer serious damage, and in the worst cases to the extent of being destroyed. When this occurs in the lungs it is likely to be diagnosed as TB or COPD (Chronic Obstructive Pulmonary Disease).

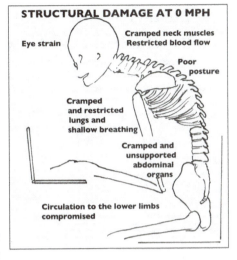

STRUCTURAL DAMAGE AT 0 MPH

Eye strain

Cramped neck muscles
Restricted blood flow

Poor posture

Cramped and restricted lungs and shallow breathing

Cramped and unsupported abdominal organs

Circulation to the lower limbs compromised

Living ribs

If your ribs have become too inactive the situation can be almost as serious. Oxygen is absorbed by the blood in your lungs, and carried throughout the body by the red blood cells, so if you are anaemic it means that these cells are deficient, potentially both in number and in quality. The result is an inadequate transportation of oxygen. Red blood cells are produced within the bone marrow, which is in the long bones of the body. The most numerous of these long bones are your ribs, and if these are allowed to become idle, their marrow-activity is depressed. In really bad cases this could mean the partial failure of your major source of red cells.

Bands of muscle that contract and extend interlink your ribs and this causes them to move together or apart. Between each rib and its neighbours there are spaces along which arteries, veins and nerves run, providing the circulation of blood to the muscles and to the marrow within the ribs. So you can see that full movement of your ribs, shoulders and arms and a relaxed but upright posture are essential for effective and full oxygenation of your whole body.

Exercises

If your breathing has been shallow for some considerable time then some other muscles might be used to re-activate your intercostal

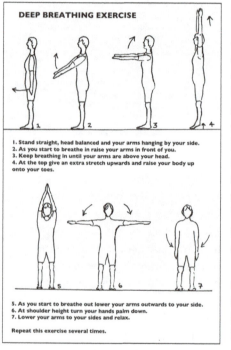

DEEP BREATHING EXERCISE

1. Stand straight, head balanced and your arms hanging by your side.
2. As you start to breathe in raise your arms in front of you.
3. Keep breathing in until your arms are above your head.
4. At the top give an extra stretch upwards and raise your body up onto your toes.

5. As you start to breathe out lower your arms outwards to your side.
6. At shoulder height turn your hands palm down.
7. Lower your arms to your sides and relax.

Repeat this exercise several times.

muscles. Your pectorals can be employed. These are the muscles between your upper arm and the front of your chest, whose function is to bring your arms downward and forward. However, if you raise your arms above your head, the pull on your pectorals lifts the ribcage upward and outward, this increases the volume in the chest cavity. When your arms are lowered the ribs collapse and the air is driven out.

So, stand comfortably upright with your arms by your sides. Start a long, steady inhalation; at the same time, bring the arms forward and upward, so that at full inspiration they are right above the head. To emphasise the point, rise on the toes and give the fingers a little extra stretch upward. Without pause, start breathing out, and lower the arms sideways until they once more hang at your sides. Making a moderate effort to keep the arms pressed back, while lowering them, effectively counters any tendency to round shoulders.

LIVE WELL. EAT WELL. BE WELL.

You can practice the above exercise at different speeds and the breathing should always be in and out through your nose. (The reasons for this will be explained later.) If you are too unwell to attempt even the lightest exercise in an upright position, a simplified version of it can be an excellent first step in the direction of more vigorous and effective breathing. You can even use the headboard of your bed to gently pull the chest wall upward. This movement helps to ease the strain on the organs in your thorax, your heart and lungs, and brings more much needed oxygen into your body.

Simple exercises to help you breathe more effectively

1 Straighten your spine. Pull your head gently back so that it balances comfortably on top of your spine, with the chin drawn in slightly, then push the crown of your head as high as you can.

2 Pull back your shoulders, but try not to raise them in the process. Try to swing your shoulder blades in behind your chest – rather than over the top towards your neck.

3 Breathe in quite steadily, and try to make the upper part of your chest open forward and sideways as the lungs fill. Let your arms hang loosely by your sides. Breathe out, and feel the ribs collapse.

4 Go for a brisk walk, breathing fully and swinging your arms freely. The arm movement activates the shoulder girdle, so applies a form of massage to the upper ribs. The walking itself will induce fuller breathing and by making an effort to draw in your stomach, the upper chest will be made to move more.

5 If walking is impossible, a simple and effective movement

– while sitting or standing still – is to take a full breath with the diaphragm then, while holding the breath, pull the tummy in. This will open out the chest quite effectively. If you are a sedentary worker, or otherwise non-active, strengthening your abdominal wall can be every bit as important to your overall health as more efficient breathing.

Breathing through your nose

There are several vital functions that the nose and its internal membranes carry out, not least warming and moistening the air entering your body before it is allowed into the deeper tubes of the respiratory system. The bony structures of the interior of the nose are also involved, and the air has to flow turbulently over a large area of mucous membrane. These are well supplied with blood vessels so that warmth and moisture are transferred to the air. This allows it to reach a state suitable for the delicate linings of windpipe and bronchial tubes. At the same time, efficient filtration of dust-particles is carried out by the moisture-covered hairs.

Effective cleansing, warming and moistening of the incoming air rely on the warmth provided by the outgoing air passing over them. In addition the cleansing function of the nasal passages must suffer if the air flow is only inward. With only incoming air the hairs become dried out, and therefore less efficient at capturing dust particles. Those arrested are likely to be dislodged by the next incoming breath and carried further into the respiratory system. With the proper alternations of direction, the hairs are kept moist and the large dust particles brought in by one inhalation have an even chance of being carried out again by a subsequent outflow of air.

Mouth breathing

For short bursts of violent exertion, adequate respiration may only be possible through mouth breathing. However, this should almost never mean breathing in through the mouth, only exhaling. It might be that you have become accustomed to an in-through-the-nose and out-through-the-mouth form of breathing; but this puts an unfair burden on your throat and bronchial tubes. Breathing in through your mouth is never really advisable, but in extreme circumstances it may be the only way. One obvious example is acute catarrhal obstruction, in which the nose is totally useless. So, with a heavy head-cold, it is sensible to avoid extremes of dryness or dustiness and to cover the mouth with thick but porous woollen cloth when the air is cold.

Outdoor exercise

If you are unfortunate enough to have to spend a great deal of your working life in an ill-ventilated room, it is imperative to get out in fresh air for considerably more than a few minutes each day. It is tantamount to cruelty to expect your body to stand up to such treatment without eventually causing serious breakdown. When they are deprived of their normal stimulus of cool, fresh air, both your skin and lungs become devitalised. The work that they are unable to accomplish will have to be shouldered by your other vital organs, and the kidneys are at immediate risk. The probability is that the body will resort to storing wastes within, laying the foundations for repeated healing crises.

Points to remember

1 Your body needs an adequate and regular supply of freshly oxygenated blood.
2 Breathing in deeply through your nose brings in fresh filtered air.
3 Breathing out fully, also through your nose, ensures that the stale air is removed and your mucous membranes are kept moist and warm.
4 Full movement of your ribs and diaphragm ensures full breathing.
5 Exercises that involve rib activity and swinging the arms are beneficial.
6 Exercise in the fresh air and a daily brisk walk will ensure a better supply of oxygen to your tissues.

LIVE WELL. EAT WELL. BE WELL.

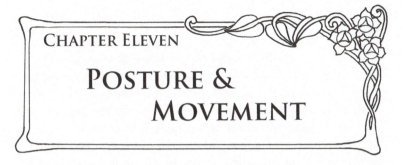

CHAPTER ELEVEN

POSTURE &
MOVEMENT

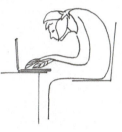

'KEEP THEM MOVING' is the first rule to avoid exacerbating a disturbance when people have gathered together in an angry crowd. So, as a parallel, within your own body any areas of congestion accompanied by a lack of movement are commonly responsible for serious disorders. Being rigid in your thinking is often mirrored in physical stiffness and inertia and is commonly at the root of many disease conditions. We often describe this situation as being 'stuck' and some significant restoration of flexibility and movement are essential for you to return to good health.

In the last chapter we looked at how your posture affects your breathing, but we also know that worry, anxiety and digestive disorders can produce excessive tension in your body. Your tense neck puts pressure on the local nerves and starts to compromise mental ability through the obstruction of the flow of the blood to your brain. Then your inability to think clearly and conclusively leads to worry, so the miserable cycle repeats, with ever-widening distressing effects on your body as a whole.

Strain

If you are a habitually worried person, this state of mind is likely to be intensified by, and may even be determined, by, your posture at work. If you are able to hold your head in a more erect position, so that it is more balanced on top of the spine, the tensions in your neck will be relieved. But, sadly, a natural, balanced posture is not often possible with many kinds of work, so the next best thing is to lift your head frequently. A rest of even a few seconds will refresh your hardest-worked muscles and allow a better flow of blood to your head.

Nerves

Another intense effect of poor working posture is the strain in your chest and upper abdomen caused by tension in your neck. The action of your heart and the early processes of digestion are controlled by your cranial nerves. Whereas the greater bulk of nerves linking the brain and the body pass through the neck safely protected within the bony 'tunnel' provided by the spinal column, these cranial nerves lie just under the surface flesh of the neck beside the muscles. This means that the cranial nerves can be exposed to prolonged pressures when a muscle is in tension. This can prevent the nervous system from being able to effectively convey messages.

A brief, light pressure, especially if repeated, may be stimulating, whereas a prolonged heavy pressure causes a numbing sensation. Too much stimulation may become irritating, but it is the unrelieved squeeze that really holds up the messages, and this can lead to disturbed heart rhythms and indigestion or heartburn.

Relaxation of the excess tensions is obviously desirable, and as with the rest of your body, the most effective relaxation is produced by doing something, usually completely different from your usual occupation. If your neck is usually stretched forwards, for instance, the aim should be to move your head backward. This can be done without any lasting discomfort if the movement is slow and steady. This latter point is important, because too many people whip their heads dizzily around when exercise is suggested and produce even greater discomfort. Try turning your head sideways to slowly and steadily look over one shoulder before turning to look straight ahead, then over the other shoulder. Bend your head from side to side, gently letting your ear move towards your shoulder on one side and repeating the movement with the other. Care should be taken to avoid lifting the shoulder to meet the ear, as this reduces the effectiveness of the exercise. Then lift your shoulders up towards your ears as you breathe in and let them drop completely as you breathe out. All the above simple exercises can help to loosen those tense neck muscles.

Regular movement

Prolonged spells in any fixed position, however comfortable it seems to be, is ultimately damaging. The key is movement, good breathing and regular changes of position and posture. If your head and neck posture is your only consideration, then try carrying things of moderate weight on your head, this at least allows you to balance your head comfortably on the top of your spine.

It seems to be a common misconception that any part of the body that is not moving is at rest, and few people have an appreciation of the sheer weight of their own head and limbs. If you are unsure about this try lifting someone's head up when they are lying down. Most of our limb movements are produced at what the physicist calls 'mechanical disadvantage', so that even

NECK EXERCISES – Do these slowly

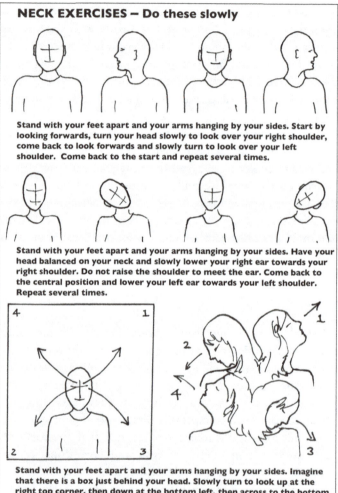

Stand with your feet apart and your arms hanging by your sides. Start by looking forwards, turn your head slowly to look over your right shoulder, come back to look forwards and slowly turn to look over your left shoulder. Come back to the start and repeat several times.

Stand with your feet apart and your arms hanging by your sides. Have your head balanced on your neck and slowly lower your right ear towards your right shoulder. Do not raise the shoulder to meet the ear. Come back to the central position and lower your left ear towards your left shoulder. Repeat several times.

Stand with your feet apart and your arms hanging by your sides. Imagine that there is a box just behind your head. Slowly turn to look up at the right top corner, then down at the bottom left, then across to the bottom right corner and up to the top left. Repeat several times.
NB: Breathe in as you relax and out as you do the stretch.

LIVE WELL. EAT WELL. BE WELL.

to hold an arm still may involve comparatively large forces. Again, if you want an illustration of this try holding your arm straight out from your shoulder, quite still, for three minutes. Very few can last that long, and only the exceptional individual can exceed it without agony or sheer willpower. Yet this involves muscular effort not much greater than we ask of our necks when we sit for hours over a desk. Similarly but on a comparatively microscopic scale, we also tend to keep certain muscles within the eyeball in a fixed state for long periods. We are surprised to develop a tired ache in the eyes when reading or looking for long periods at a computer screen. The outstretched arm experiment should help to explain the reason for your discomfort.

Cramp and spasms

Any muscle that is in action, in the sense of exerting its pull, is consuming nutrients and oxygen and producing wastes. If the former two are not replaced as they are used up, and the latter removed immediately, strength wanes and pain begins. The blood-stream is responsible for carrying fresh materials to the tissues and wastes away from them. Muscle movement of limbs and trunk assist the circulation. The mechanism depends upon the presence of a multitude of non-return valves within the veins. In many everyday occupations, bits of your body are held motionless or used for repetitive movements for many minutes, sometimes hours, at a time. In this situation your circulation in a whole area tends to become deficient.

The first sign is tiredness, gradually developing into a real ache, and eventually becoming cramp. These are graduating stages in the accumulation of acid wastes within your muscles. At this point the muscle fibres go into full contraction. There are manifold reasons for cramp or muscle spasms to occur; occasionally small muscles go into protective spasm and these rapid muscle shortenings can be very painful, though often their action is to protect distressed nerve or other muscle tissue nearby. Whatever the reason for your cramp or spasm they are much less likely to occur when your diet is sufficiently supplied with all the necessary vitamins, trace elements and minerals and your bloodstream is clean, your circulation is free and your limbs and trunk are being used actively in a truly natural range of movements.

Keep moving

Whether we like it or not, our arms move when we walk. This is claimed to be a relic of our ancestral mode of locomotion, when our ancestors ran around safely balanced on four legs, instead of rather precariously on two. Our arms are often prevented from swinging by carrying a heavy suitcase or fully laden supermarket bags. These unnatural occupations put unrelieved strain on the neck and shoulder area, and keep your arm muscles in a state of constant tension. Fortunately, most of us become so uncomfortable that we change our position fairly often, but there can be delayed pain in the muscles that have been too long in unrelieved contraction. The lack of movement in the arms also denies the ribs that helpful pull to greater movement. As we explored in the last chapter, for an ample production of red blood cells, there must be continual activity of the ribcage, as well as space within the chest for full lung expansion and for the heart to beat freely.

The abdomen

One of the heaviest tasks that your abdominal muscles have to do is help support your intestines, and this is in addition to what should be their primary work. If you are fit and healthy, your intestines should be supported principally by internal structures, and your abdominal muscles are there to assist the movement of your body. Strong abdominal muscles are produced by strong exercise, and if the aim is to restore strength it is essential to exercise in the right way. Unless the exercises are remedial, they can very easily aggravate an already serious condition. If your intestines have started to sag, any increase in pressure produced by contracting your abdominal muscles is likely to add to the downward trend. The floor of the pelvis must then take greater weight, and this can add pressure to such important parts as the nerves and blood vessels that supply your legs and the pelvic organs. It is for this reason that we mainly recommend that when you start doing abdominal exercises that you attempt them while in an inverted position. Gravity then helps to pull your intestines toward the diaphragm and away from your pelvis, this in turn allows the lower areas of the abdominal wall to contract more effectively. The inversion may be comparatively mild, as produced by lying on an abdominal board, this doesn't need to be an expensive piece of kit, a wide plank with one end raised about 20–30 cm off the floor will suffice. Make sure that it is secure and will not move when you start to lie on it, with your feet high and your head low. As you become more fit and able you should be able to progress to true inverted poses with only head, shoulders and elbows on the floor. In this position you can do 'scissors', 'cycling' and 'striding' movements.

Avoid the much over-rated exercise of trying to touch your toes, it is quite useless as a remedial movement if you have weak abdominal muscles and can add to the strain on already distressed tissues. Also remember that it is the posture in which your heaviest movements are made that tend to become fixed, so it is important

SLANT PLANK AND FLOOR EXERCISES

Prop your plank up securely on a solid rise. Lie on the plank with your feet raised and allow your abdominal organs to settle into place, relax and let your lumbar spine drop towards the plank

Steady youself with your arms on the floor. Bend your knees up and pull your pelvic floor muscles up towards your stomach. Hold this for a few seconds and then relax. Repeat this several times before straightening your legs again

As you gain confidence raise one leg straight up, engaging your stomach muscles, then raise the other leg. Lower your legs one at a time. As you get stronger try to raise both legs at the same time. Pausing on the way up and on the way down will give a stronger pull on your stomach muscles

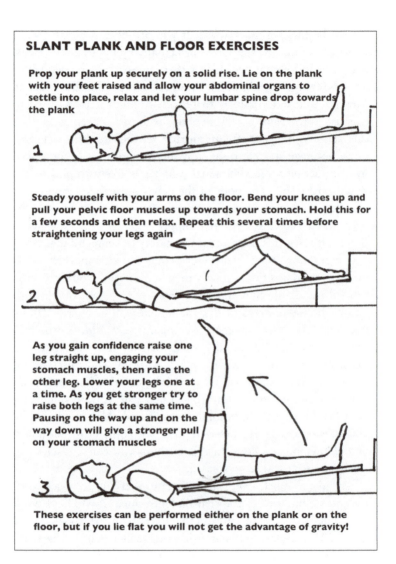

These exercises can be performed either on the plank or on the floor, but if you lie flat you will not get the advantage of gravity!

LIVE WELL. EAT WELL. BE WELL.

to avoid heavy work in a cramped, stooped or otherwise constricting posture.

Garments designed to help support your weak abdomen may give you a better appearance but are more likely to further weaken your natural structures and add to your internal discomfort. Instead, as often as you can throughout the day, use your abdominal muscles to attempt to pull the contents of your abdomen up from the pelvis towards your chest. At first there may be only a token response, but gradually the control should improve. The great thing is that you can practice this exercise anywhere, anytime. This muscular effort can be complemented by a cold Squat Splash in the mornings – best taken immediately after you have performed your inverted exercise. Run three to four inches of really cold (not tepid) water into the bath; squat down with only your toes immersed then scoop handfuls of water alternately and vigorously on to the abdomen and between the legs. An alternative to this is to use a flexible shower-head and direct the spray to the same areas; adjusting the flow until a comfortable level is reached. There is more detailed information about this in the chapter 'Water and Nature Cure'.

The spinal column

For some reason when we exercise we tend to forget about the spine. It is too often regarded as a mere 'backbone' for the rest of your skeletal structure, without any real articulation or movements of its own. Most of the spinal column's many units in the lumbar, thoracic and cervical sections should each be able to articulate smoothly with their neighbours above and below. In this way the correct relationships are preserved, persistent strains are avoided and the flows of blood and nervous energy are unimpeded. With limited or one-sided movement, fibrous thickenings may take the place of active muscle and intolerable pressures can develop on the softer tissues of the column. Gross deformity of the spine may be uncommon, but distorted curves accompanied by loss of mobility are to be found everywhere.

To encourage normal flexibility in the spinal column, a simple yet effective exercise consists of grasping any support above your head, and then you need to swing your body in wide, circular sweeps, so that the spine is successively curved in each direction. Requiring a little more effort, but without any apparatus, are the ordinary trunk-bending and trunk-twisting movements. These are made more effective by extending the arms and performing them firmly and steadily so that the leverage carries the movement a little beyond the gentler limits. Please keep in mind the earlier caution about excessive forward bending.

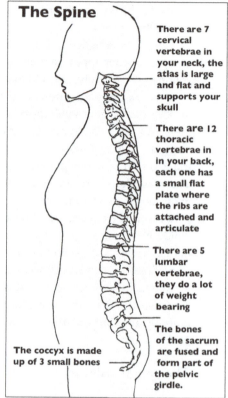

The Spine

There are 7 cervical vertebrae in your neck, the atlas is large and flat and supports your skull

There are 12 thoracic vertebrae in in your back, each one has a small flat plate where the ribs are attached and articulate

There are 5 lumbar vertebrae, they do a lot of weight bearing

The bones of the sacrum are fused and form part of the pelvic girdle.

The coccyx is made up of 3 small bones

LIVE WELL. EAT WELL. BE WELL.

Legs

It will be obvious from what has already been discussed that the majority of us simply do not use our legs nearly enough and this can be exacerbated by the habit of sitting with your legs crossed at the knee. This has several deleterious effects, of which pelvic strain and obstructed circulation are probably the most obvious. In some cases, knee-crossing is indicative of emotional distress, and the individual who twines one leg around the other can often be discontent about their relationship to life. It is essentially a gesture of insecurity or defensiveness, and adopting such a strong self-protecting posture is not necessarily the best way to face the world.

Walking, as we constantly bang on about, is an excellent exercise, but it is worth selecting your route with some thought. Walking along hard roads with dead flat surfaces may cause more damage to, rather than improve, an existing devitalised condition of the legs and feet. Also the fumes that you are likely to breathe in from the passing traffic will not help your oxygen levels. From a simply muscular point of view there is not enough variation in the range and position of the many muscles in the kinetic chain that runs from your toes up to your pelvis when walking on such surfaces.

For the greatest range of suitable muscle movement, walks should be taken over ground that is uneven and at least a little yielding. This activity involves continued and active readjustments of your muscles and skeleton, not only in the feet and legs, but also in the pelvis and within the spinal column. Walking on turfy ground may seem much more of an effort than on tarmac for the first mile or so, but thereafter the situation changes drastically; on grass, there is a feeling of greater vigour, while on tarmac fatigue begins to set in.

If you are in a situation where your occupation involves prolonged standing, the strain in your legs can be considerably eased by what we call 'elephant standing' – taking the weight of the body alternately on each leg, with a slow, rhythmic rocking movement. This need not be in any way obvious to the casual onlooker, and can be further improved by rolling over on to the outer edge of each foot in turn, curling the toes inside the shoes while doing so. Such simple routines can keep fatigue away for hours, and are positively helpful in assisting the circulation and keeping the arches of the feet in good condition.

The feet

In the horse world there is a very old saying 'No foot, no horse'. It may sound a bit drastic, but the damage that can be done to your feet and the entire skeletal and muscular balance of your body by wearing unsuitable footwear is far reaching. Inappropriate shoes can completely nullify the possible benefits of walking, by producing rigidity and cramping. The wearing of high heels imbalances the lower leg muscles and causes the lumbar spine to adopt an unnatural inward carriage, known as lordosis.

Ideally shoes should be flat and your toes should be free to spread as they take your body's weight, your big toe should be pointing straight ahead so that it can take its proper and vital part in forming a strong elastic bridge to support you. Good quality and well-designed trainers are possibly the best option provided they are made of breathable materials. Go barefoot or in stockinged feet whenever possible. Wriggle your toes actively and often. For more positive revitalisation, walking barefoot on dewy morning grass is possible for the lucky few. For others, the urban substitute is 'running on the spot' in an inch or two of cold water in the bath for one minute, this can be a part of your morning exercises and cold splash.

The mind

Someone once said: 'The mind is like a parachute; it only works when it's open'. We have too often found that rigidity in thinking is one aspect of a widespread inclination that many people have to get things 'right' and then refuse to change. This chapter opened with an observation on how resistance to change can set up all sorts of tensions and inflexibilities in your body. Even Nature Cure practitioners can, of course, sympathise with this fear of change. The stresses we all face in modern life can seem overwhelming, changes come so frequently and quickly and we are bombarded by 24-hour news and instant messaging. However, a refusal to embrace change, or at least investigate it, can lead to a reduced enjoyment of life and a feeling of being left behind.

The process of adding to your knowledge should be enjoyable; you could even make it an aim to learn something new every day. Greater understanding of the situations and events that most affect your life can help you to develop your views, and your growing confidence will in turn enable you to deal with all manner of problems you will encounter. To accept a method or answer as being 'right' for all time is to deny the possibility of progress

There are many situations in life where there is genuinely no escape from a choice between two unacceptable options. An open and flexible mind will be able to assess those choices and opt for the more ethical, or the least unethical, course, while the closed mind can easily be flummoxed. But having made the choice, it is essential to remember why you took it and to continue to move forward in the right direction.

Read, listen, learn and expand your knowledge, keep what makes sense to you in your situation and don't be afraid to discard what doesn't. Build your own individual approach to your life, if it works for you, and keeps you truly healthy; don't be afraid to follow that course. Always with the proviso, of course, that your chosen path causes no harm to your fellow humans and other animals. The interesting thing is that when we choose the more honest and healthiest way, it is often also the kindest option for our shared planet.

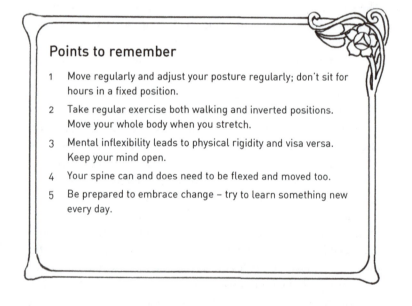

Points to remember

1 Move regularly and adjust your posture regularly; don't sit for hours in a fixed position.

2 Take regular exercise both walking and inverted positions. Move your whole body when you stretch.

3 Mental inflexibility leads to physical rigidity and visa versa. Keep your mind open.

4 Your spine can and does need to be flexed and moved too.

5 Be prepared to embrace change – try to learn something new every day.

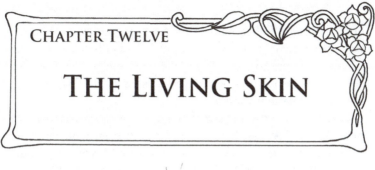

CHAPTER TWELVE

THE LIVING SKIN

SO FAR WE have been looking at the internal structures of our body, now we will take a brief look at the importance of our largest organ, the skin.

We are all aware of the importance of our skin to our appearance – showing us to be either rosy cheeked and glowing with health or 'pale and interesting'. Too often we cover our skin in cosmetics in a vain attempt to alter the way we look and smell, and the way we feel about ourselves, yet our health actually depends heavily on our skin's activity. When a Nature Cure practitioner checks the state of the blood cleansing organs of a new patient, the skin is first on the list. Not only does its superficial position make it easy to examine, its condition reflects that of the body as a whole.

The strength and activity of your skin depends on the nourishment it receives. Most of the expensively advertised cosmetics, that claim to nourish the skin, add nothing genuinely constructive, but the rubbing in that is an essential part of their application can be quite effective. Any lotions, creams, salves or balms, no matter whether they are based on so called 'natural' ingredients or on a chemical cocktail, only weaken your skin in the long run by lowering its natural vitality.

The water content of your skin not only affects its appearance but also its elasticity. If you are suffering from fluid retention (oedema) you skin is likely to look puffy and it will not rapidly reform after being stretched. Instead of springing back into shape, the distended area tends to fill with fluid that makes it heavy and opaque. This effect can be seen in most parts of your body, but perhaps most obviously around your face, wrists and ankles. Those 'bags under your eyes' and swelling around the joints are pointers towards an inner ill-health.

The elasticity and tone of your skin are important to how you look, but these factors are really much more vitally involved with its protective functions. If you skin is healthy it can absorb some heavy blows without tearing or even showing more than a slight bruising afterwards. It yields just enough to accept the energy of the impact, yet not so much as to allow the underlying tissues and organs to be harmed. The healthier your skin, the greater its tensile strength and toughness; skin that is retaining fluid has only a fraction of the strength which characterises its drier state. A lack of toughness can be betrayed by a tendency to bruise with even the slightest impact. If you bruise easily and cuts take too long to heal, attention to your diet and exercise routines is needed.

Speedy healing

Reducing your intake of liquids of all kinds, in particular those with an active ingredient, such as tea, coffee and alcoholic drinks, and avoiding junk foods and instead eating more fresh raw foods are first essentials. Occasionally, Nature Cure followers have to undergo surgical operations for the repair of physical defects, or as the result of accidental injury, and it is gratifying how often the surgeon remarks to such a patient that the tissues were unusually firm and the healing remarkably rapid. A healthy, living skin should be as tough as the best leather, and over much of the body human skin is at least as thick as, for example, the leather overalls worn by motorcyclists.

Skin and regulation of temperature

Regulating the body's temperature is probably one of the most critical functions of your skin. If it fails in this task, even for quite a short time, you will be unable to maintain many of your vital activities. The human body is enabled to work efficiently largely because its conditions are standardised, kept in homeostasis. To a great extent, your body temperature is controlled by the amount of heat generated inside it, and this is a matter for the internal organs and controls; but when heat production is either limited by shortage of fuel or greatly augmented by heavy muscular activity, it is your skin which must compensate promptly and effectively.

Two factors work together in this process; the speed of the flow of blood through the surface vessels, and the dampness of the skin. When the vessels are kept tiny, by the constricting effect of the muscles that surround them, and the skin is dry, there is very little heat loss. Your skin may feel quite cold, but your deeper organs are still kept warm enough to stop them becoming chilled. But when there is excessive internal heat production the surface blood vessels dilate and the blood flows through them rapidly; this initiates an almost simultaneous increase in perspiration, and a great deal of excess heat can be lost in a very short time.

Exercise vitally important

The prompt and effective operation of these measures depends on the alertness of your skin, which in turn depends on its physical activity. Over-protecting your skin can lower the speed and efficiency of the responses. Your skin is kept in good condition by being used, and used hard. To isolate the skin from sudden changes in temperature, such as it would encounter in more natural conditions is to lower its ability to respond quickly. A quick change in temperature will produce a correspondingly vigorous reaction in the sentinels and regulators – the sensory and the motor nerve fibres.

To encourage and restore the natural alertness of the skin, exposure to cold air and water are both simple and effective. The healthy reaction to a short exposure to cold air or water stimulates heat-production and we emphasise that the application should be brief. The cold splash was touched on in the last chapter and it is only necessary to repeat that any applications should be in a reasonably warm bathroom, and be followed with a vigorous towel or hand rub to dry yourself.

Throwing out wastes

Of the four cleansing organs of your body, your skin is the largest. Its task is to throw out moisture, oily waste and volatile acids. If necessary, the skin can handle increased amounts of gaseous and dissolved wastes without showing any sign of strain – although the unusual activity may be evident in other ways, such as some level of body odour. In this case washing with soap of any kind will have practically no effect on the causes of these odours; these lie in the failure of the other internal organs to deal with their tasks efficiently obliging the skin to take more than its fair share.

When this happens you must help the skin any way that you can, and something as apparently benign as long hot baths can severely restrict its effective function. Even if you do nothing more to improve the situation, activating the skin with cold splashes and rubs, and wearing light, natural silk, cotton or cellular underwear will help to remove some of the immediate vital distress.

In more serious cases, the acid wastes handled by the skin are too concentrated, and some level of inflammation occurs. In the orthodox approach this would be called a 'skin disease', but it is the whole body that is diseased; your skin is simply doing its best to make it less so. Here again, allowing the waste matter to escape as freely as possible can help to minimise the distress, and frequent washing with cool or cold water may be helpful. But this really is a matter for attention to your whole way of life, skin eruptions are as likely to be caused by emotional factors as dietary errors.

Skin 'infections'

Sometimes, the skin throws out wastes that do not appear to cause noticeable irritation, but that, unless removed rapidly, provide excellent conditions for the growth of microorganisms. If these are bacterial, as in impetigo, their proliferation is put down to either staphylococcus or streptococcus 'infecting' skin already damaged for instance from a scratch or a graze. If it is fungal, as in ringworm or athlete's foot, collectively known as tinea, then this type of growth tends to enjoy warm moist areas of the body. The diagnosis is not fundamental, and in both cases it is customary to blame the infection on outside factors. But the sad truth is that had your skin not been in an unhealthy state to begin with there

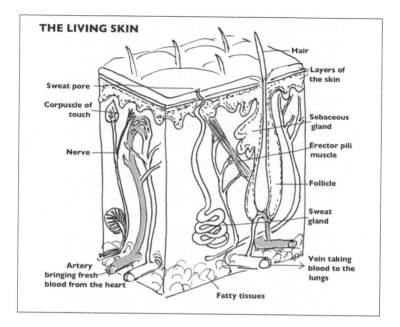

THE LIVING SKIN

Hair

Layers of the skin

Sweat pore

Corpuscle of touch

Sebaceous gland

Erector pili muscle

Nerve

Follicle

Sweat gland

Vein taking blood to the lungs

Artery bringing fresh blood from the heart

Fatty tissues

would have been no 'culture medium' for the visitors to multiply upon. Frequent changes of underclothing and a liberal use of non-bacterial non-perfumed soapy water are helpful for local relief, but cutting out rich, sweet, processed non-foods is far more important in the long run.

Surface condition

Maintenance of the skin's outer surface is normally performed by the production of numerous layers of cells, which become flattened (squamous) as they are pressed outward by the newer ones beneath. A short distance below the surface, the cells cease to be nourished and die, forming a layer of tough, inert 'leather'. Since this surface would be rapidly broken up by friction, bending and wetting, it has to be kept lubricated and more or less waterproof. One greasy secretion that does this is called sebum, and is produced by the sebaceous glands – one at the root of each hair. In addition, some of the greasy wastes thrown out by the sweat glands are temporarily re-absorbed into the surface. They are eventually lost when the surface is worn away in the normal course of everyday life.

Often, we hear complaints of 'dry skin' but this is not always due to deficiency of lubricant. There may be an excessive acid secretion which approaches eczematous concentrations, and which makes the skin hard and scaly. Sometimes, this sub-eczema is more noticeable as a slight stickiness, but in either case there will be other symptoms of acidosis. In cold weather particularly, however, it is lack of lubricant that is principally responsible. When the circulation near the surface is restricted for long periods, the glandular activity almost ceases and the greases are worn or washed away faster than they are replaced.

Avoid olive oil

For immediate relief, any inert greasy substance applied to the skin is helpful. Probably the safest is simple lanolin, which is nothing more than the same kind of grease as should be present naturally, but produced by a sheep. As it is usually only on the back of your hands that get really dry the occasional use of a small amount on the affected area is fine. Any topical treatment creams should be used sparingly, as ever, as the more you do for your body the less it will do for itself. However, do not use olive oil; this might seem to be the most harmless of all, but olive oil is not stable. That is, it breaks down rapidly, producing fatty acids that can irritate the deeper, living layers of the skin. Even if this does not occur, the nourishing nature of olive oil is highly attractive to microorganisms, and there is no sense in creating a suitable habitat for them.

Protective powers

The protective function of your skin is not limited to mechanical assaults. There are many things, living and inorganic, in the environment generally, which could rapidly destroy your tissues if they reached them. The waterproof top layer of your skin keeps most things out; rain, dust and other assorted particles in the atmosphere, and all manner of substances that we handle in our daily work. We can even scoop up many kinds of chemicals in our bare hands – substances that would cause violent poisoning if either injected through a cut or swallowed in minute quantities. Such everyday substances as sugar and salt can be destructive if they reach an open wound, but are harmless on a whole skin if they are dry and not kept too long in contact with it.

Those who accept the Nature Cure teachings about the causes of disease, but still have a lingering superstition about the malevolent power of germs, may be further reassured by the fact that a healthy skin is probably the most powerful germicide known. More research in 2012 by teams in the University of Pennsylvania and the National Institute of Allergy and Infectious Diseases in Maryland have both shown that there is a strong likelihood that a healthy population of non-pathogenic skin microbes, now known as the 'microbiome', act as a barrier against pathogenic microbes trying to gain a toehold in your skin.

Sterilising stupidities

One way of reducing the skin's natural resistance to invasion is to slosh a strong antiseptic over it whenever a minor scratch or cut is sustained. Iodine used to be the chemical of choice and was probably responsible for more slow healing wounds and unnecessarily large scars than any other form of mistaken treatment. Today you can take your pick. Just search the Internet for an antiseptic and you can have it as spray, a liquid or a cream. Killing many millions of cells in the vicinity, when some thousands have already been damaged by injury is merely to multiply the problem. Washing the wound with clean water is helpful to the body, but sterilising a whole area by chemical poisoning is not.

Another way of undermining the protective function of our skin, and one which is unhappily increasing, is to remove the natural oils with synthetic detergents. Soap is not a natural product, but its efficiency as a remover of surplus grease is just about as much as the human skin can, and should have to, stand on a regular basis. The newer synthetics go far beyond soap in seeking out and making soluble the greases in the skin, and complications are only to be expected. The latest craze for antibacterial hand washes in the home can only add to the burden, they are not 'selective weed killers' and there is no doubt they will kill as many of the vital 'good' germs as the 'baddies'.

Caution with detergents

Unfortunately, you do not have to immerse yourself, or even just your hands, in detergent-containing washing-up water to acquire a significant coating of the stuff. More than a trace remains adherent to clothing which has been washed in it, even after repeated rinsings. Take care with your choice of laundry liquids and powders and avoid the biological types. If you are prone to skin conditions preferably wash your underwear by hand using a simple soap and rinse well until the water runs clear. Apart from the irritant effect of the detergents themselves – and we hear many reports of acute and lasting misery from this cause – there is the concomitant reduced resistance to other foreign substances. There are various skin conditions that can have their origin in the irritant effects of detergents. These include reddened skin, scaly patches, blistering, burning or itching, swelling around the eyes, face and genitals or even the whole body, hives, darkened leathery skin and sun sensitivity. So it is well worth finding the right washing products, or you could even invest in some laundry balls that allow you to wash a load without any detergents at all.

Sunlight and vitamins

Sunbathing as a healthy pastime goes in and out of fashion with each successive research finding, however the value of ultra-violet light to the growing child and to adults in sensible amounts was never in question. Sadly sunbathing is currently regarded as a 'dangerous' pastime, mainly, in our view, as a direct result of the use of sun blocks and sun creams. Instead of the body being able to warn of excessive ultraviolet by responding with erythema – painful reddening of the skin – people are staying out in the sun for far too long believing that they are protected. The ultimate penalty is being paid, particularly amongst the fair-skinned of the Northern Hemisphere, who choose to holiday in sunnier climes, in the form of skin cancer. You need exposure to sunshine to be healthy, and patients at Kingston had access to sunbathing enclosures in the grounds and there was also the careful use of

LIVE WELL. EAT WELL. BE WELL.

sun-ray lamps in the short winter days. My grandfather gained the nickname The Sunshine Doctor when he set up his practice in Edinburgh on his return to Scotland and early Nature Cure followers were ridiculed and reviled for claiming that there was any benefit at all in sunlight. This was echoed in the way in which they were scoffed at for telling people that fresh vegetables were an important part of a healthy diet. Early naturopaths were well aware of the existence and significance of what they called the 'living elements' of fresh food which were later, and orthodoxly, renamed 'vitamins'.

So what has sunshine to do with vitamins?

Ultraviolet (UVB) light falling on the skin is absorbed by it, and synthesised into active compounds known collectively as Vitamin D. Passing into the bloodstream, the vitamin is carried through the body, and takes part in vital processes wherever calcium is being handled. This occurs most actively in the bones of growing children and in older people it aids tissue repair, but we all need it to keep healthy. Without vitamin D, the body cannot make proper use of calcium, and the structures that normally contain much of this element become weakened and deformed. Vitamin D naturally occurs in oily fish and eggs, otherwise it is from the sun. Even a small exposed area such as the face and hands may be quite adequate for an adult if there is much sunlight, but this is scarcely enough for a growing child. Sadly rickets has made an unwelcome return recently according to the NHS. Those who naturally have more melatonin in their skin need longer in the sun to achieve the same level of vitamin D in their systems than those of fairer skin colouring. To quote from their website:

Other groups who are at risk are children born prematurely and children taking medication that interferes with vitamin D. However, any child whose diet does not contain enough vitamin D or calcium can develop rickets.[1]

Add to this list the child who is no longer allowed to play outside in the sunshine, because of perceived risks from strangers, traffic and, of course, the sun!

In a varied diet, containing a moderate amount of dairy produce, some of the body's needs of the vitamin are provided in 'tangible' form, but the modern fad for adding synthetic or concentrate vitamin D to almost any processed food is quite unreliable. Many authorities are becoming seriously concerned about the increasing evidence of problems arising from an excess of the artificial version given to infants and children, either by their parents or as 'welfare' supplements. An excess of Vitamin D can cause hypervitaminosis D, this can cause a build up of calcium in the blood and damage to the liver and kidneys. So it's best to get your Vitamin D from the sun, but in sensible doses.

Protective pigments

It is equally possible, of course, to receive too much sunlight, and to suffer accordingly, but this has automatic compensations that are lacking from the synthetic substances. For one thing, the blood can 'take it or leave it' if an unnecessarily large amount of vitamin D is formed in the skin, but the bowel does not seem to have the same ability when fats saturated with the chemical are presented to it. Secondly, the same rays that form the vitamin also stimulate the production of pigment in the skin, so prolonged exposure to sunlight causes a yellow-brown colouring to appear, varying in individual cases from a few pale freckles to a deep tan. This yellowy pigment absorbs the ultra-violet light strongly, so that less penetrates to the layers where the vitamin would be formed and absorbed.

Sunbathing, then, should be carried out with intelligence. If you have naturally fair skin quite short exposures will provide adequate irradiation. With a darker skin, much longer exposures can be comfortably tolerated, and are often necessary to obtain an equivalent benefit.

Feedback

Our skin is richly provided with nerve-endings. Apart from the sense organs, your skin has a more intensive system of detection than any other structure of the body. Our civilised clothing deprives us of much of the sensation we should otherwise experience. Civilised or not, there are very few days when many of us would venture out without clothing or even leave our waterproofs at home. Mostly it is only our faces and hands that are in contact with the atmosphere, and it is through them that we are able to appreciate the sun's warmth in early spring, the feel of rain on our faces or the cutting bite of a chill wind. The greatly intensified sensation that can be experienced when larger areas of skin are exposed is the joy of sun, water and air bathing. It is through these experiences that we get a real idea of the truer impact of the environment around us than at any time in our normal workaday life. This heightened awareness can do nothing but good; the sensations are natural and invigorating, reminding us that the real world is a far more substantial and alive thing than the artificial world of computer games and news feeds.

The sensitivity and reliability of your skin's feedback depend to a large extent on the amount of use it receives as well as the distribution and density of nerve endings. Surfaces that we use often – and, interestingly, more so if we can see them in action – develop an acuity and precision that is quite lacking from less-used areas. The fingers, for instance, can distinguish remarkably fine detail – think of the small size of Braille characters – while your back is hardly able to distinguish the position, or even the number of points of contact, when widely-spaced fingers are placed upon it. Similarly, the face and hands are highly sensitive to thermal changes, and the heat distribution of the whole body may be altered by their feedback. Cold water on the face can relieve congestion and tension in the chest – a useful tip for those whose breathing tends to 'jam up' occasionally – while on a hot day a similar application to the wrists can produce almost the same refreshing effect as a cold drink. This can mean that you avoid taking in excessive amounts of extra liquid.

The deeper layers are alive

Wherever your skin is subjected to regular continuous heavy pressure, it tends to form a much thicker layer. The irritation stimulates the multiplication of the cells, while the external pressure may prevent the usual rapid loss from the surface. Such calluses are normally found as pads on your heels, soles and the undersurfaces of your toes. Similar pads may be formed on any part of the hand or fingers that receives intense pressure or hard wear continually. Painful corns can be formed on the feet from ill-fitting shoes, these thickenings of the skin have no option but to grow inwards and it is this in-growth that causes the pain as the tip of the corn impinges on nerves in the foot.

Moles and blotches

Moles are areas in which relatively large amounts of browny pigment – melanin – have been deposited in flat, hard platelets. This pigment is really a waste product, and its continued presence in the body is usually tolerated only in the skin. Congenital moles – or the development of a few over many years of life – have no particular significance, but a too rapid development of many moles or a radical change to the shape and size of an existing mole suggests that the body is producing and retaining too much waste of a potentially disturbing nature. You would be advised to examine your way of living and see whether changes are called for. If you have any doubts consult your Nature Cure practitioner.

The red or purple blotches that indicate over-distended capillary vessels are, like varicose veins, liable to respond only slowly to treatment and to remain partially abnormal no matter what is done. However, stimulating the area of skin involved can result in some improvement. The nervous controls will then keep the vessels in better tone – in a more contracted state – so that there is less discolouration, while an improvement to your general health should make for better oxygenation and circulation, so that the colour is clearer.

The living skin

To recap: In all its activities, your skin works best when kept busy, being subjected to all sorts of variation and handling difficult situations. It is weakened by pampering, deadened by kindness and potentially poisoned by attempts to 'feed' it from the outside. It likes to meet the elements in as natural a way as possible. When it throws waste out, it prefers to do so completely and effectively. It loves to have its surface massaged, scratched and rubbed.

What is doesn't appreciate is having its normal excretory routes clogged up with aluminium containing antiperspirants. If you are eating a reasonable diet your sweat will not be smelly and the use of these products will become unnecessary. There is research that suggests that the use of these cosmetics can cause breast cancers and dementia. Women who shave their armpits before applying antiperspirants are at greater risk than men whose hair helps to stop the absorption of the aluminium salts.

In our attempts to isolate our skins from the bumps, tickles, scorches, scratches, tingles, stings, chills, roughnesses, smoothnesses, soakings, searings, itchings and soothings which it should normally experience, we risk cutting ourselves off from the realities of life. Variety provides stimulation, and a well used skin will remain alert and ready to take whatever action it needs to meet any given situation.

It is more than coincidence that the owners of such skin will also be equally alert and interested in the world around them.

Reference

1 NHS website. www.nhs.uk

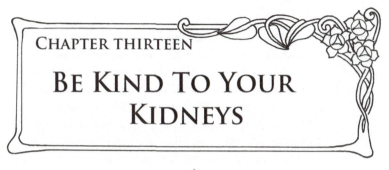

CHAPTER THIRTEEN

BE KIND TO YOUR KIDNEYS

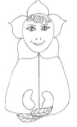

OFTEN PATIENTS WILL consult their Nature Cure practitioner because they are suffering from a skin irritation, some form of respiratory distress or perhaps a nagging headache. The main presenting symptom may be rheumatic or an apparently cardiac distress. Even if it is none of the above, we would still consider it an essential part of any preliminary consultation to assess the efficiency of your kidneys. Only rarely are these organs exempt from your overall bodily disease, yet new patients will express mild surprise, if not downright incredulity, when we suggest that the state of their kidneys is an important factor in their condition.

We are usually less interested in what your kidneys are doing than in what they are failing to do. In many cases the health of your kidneys is reflected in changes to the texture, colour and formation of your skin and underlying tissues. Urinalysis can be informative and to take two extreme instances, in Patient A it is possible for urine to be normal in composition, yet the body as a whole is showing all the signs of uraemia – a failure to excrete completely the major wastes from the bloodstream. While in Patient B the urine contains all manner of abnormal substances, yet the bodily tissues are in good condition. In the first example, the kidneys themselves may be seriously deficient in action, whereas in the second they are likely to be perfectly sound, but are being required to work much harder than normal to compensate.

Fair play

There are four sets of cleansing organs which share the burden of removing wastes from your bloodstream: your skin, lungs, liver and kidneys. When all of these are working normally there is co-ordinated action and each one does its fair share of the work. But if any one of the organs fails in its tasks, then the other three must come under more pressure. So it is that we often find the major symptom of kidney weakness to be respiratory difficulty, or sometimes an unhealthy skin. Your heart also has close affinities with kidney function and when your bloodstream is carrying too much acidic waste it becomes less fluid and more viscous, this throws a greater load on your heart and the usual response is a marked increase in blood pressures.

What the kidneys are

The kidneys are a pair of glands – each about the same size as the palm of your hand – situated just under the diaphragm on either side of the spinal column. Blood is pumped into the kidneys at full pressure from the main artery of the trunk, and the kidneys filter the blood by the action of tiny twisted tubes (called glomeruli) – of

THE LOCATION OF THE KIDNEYS

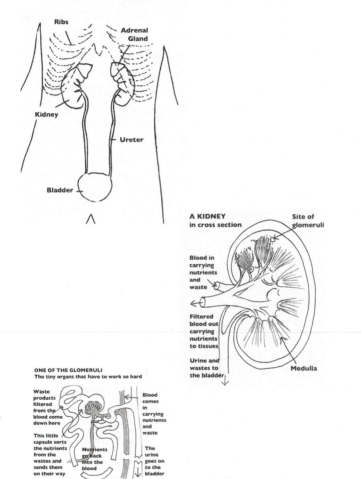

Ribs

Adrenal
Gland

Kidney

Ureter

Bladder

A KIDNEY
in cross section

Site of
glomeruli

Blood in
carrying
nutrients
and
waste

Filtered
blood out
carrying
nutrients
to tissues

Urine and
wastes to
the bladder

Medulla

ONE OF THE GLOMERULI
The tiny organs that have to work so hard

Waste
products
filtered
from the
blood come
down here

This little
capsule sorts
the nutrients
from the
wastes and
sends them
on their way

Nutrients
go back
into the
blood

Blood
comes
in
carrying
nutrients
and
waste

The
urine
goes on
to the
bladder

which there are estimated to be about one million in each kidney. At the start of each tubule is a microscopic knot of blood-vessels and a proportion of the fluid part of the blood seeps through. The remainder of the fluid part, together with the corpuscles, passes onward and out of the kidneys through veins and back into the general circulation. The fluid in the tubule then passes through and as it does so the walls re-absorb the main proportion of the substances dissolved in the liquid.

So, at the start of the tube the fluid contains both wastes and useful materials, but during transit the useful materials are taken back into the body, leaving only the surplus water and the wastes to continue on. The outpourings of the tubules are collected in funnel-shaped vessels that run together and drain into the ureter, the main pipeline to the bladder, where the urine collects until it is convenient to dispose of it.

Liquid excess

This is rather different from the popularly imagined action of the kidneys. The well-known phrase *'flushing out the kidneys'* gives a false impression of what goes on in these much-misunderstood organs. The normal surplus of fluid required for optimal functioning is supplied by a diet composed mainly of 70 per cent fresh fruit, salads and vegetables, which also provide the organised minerals and vitamins essential to all your normal healthy bodily functions.

When there is too much fluid flowing through the tubes, the kidneys' absorbent cells have to work more swiftly and more efficiently if the body is not to lose valuable materials. For the majority of us in the western world who eat a diet deficient in fresh whole foods, the result is a combination of overwork and inefficiency in the kidneys. So, far from being helpful activity, taking an excess of liquid not only upsets your digestion, assimilation and bowel efficiency, it also over-burdens your kidneys. Twice the volume of urine but half the waste removed.

Overwork

In serious cases, there are clear indications of malfunctioning of overworked kidneys in the urine in the form of particles and substances that are the results of cell breakdown. There is often tenderness in the small of the back that is the classical backache of distressed kidneys. Although the total working capacity of the kidneys is claimed to be at least four times that required in a normally healthy system it is reasonable for you to deduce that 'fair wear and tear' in the kidneys is no cause for alarm. But, no matter how great the reserves of the kidneys, those reserves have a purpose; they enable a proportion of the functional tissues to rest, recuperate and be repaired while others carry on the vital activity.

Generally, the less specialised a cell, the more easily can it be replaced if it is destroyed or removed, but the more specialised its function the more likely it is to be irreplaceable. Although all cells have normal powers of self-repair, once destroyed a very specialised cell cannot be compensated for by multiplication of adjacent cells.

Among everyday factors that are capable of destroying kidney cells are phosphoric acid – an ingredient found in many popular carbonated drinks – and several antibiotics, anticonvulsants and non-steroidal anti-inflammatory drugs (NSAIDs). Phosphoric acid can occur naturally in damaging concentrations as a result of over-eating eggs, which is why we recommend that you eat no more than 2–3 eggs per week as part of a balanced diet. Among the drugs, the antibiotic sulphonamides have a particularly vicious record. Over-consumption of alcohol can also take its toll. In more general ways, destruction of kidney cells can result from overwork combined with malnutrition. Only rarely do we find overwork alone producing vital breakdown, but when there is also lack of balance in nutrition, with the potential for a total absence of vital elements, some level of breakdown is inevitable.

What you can do about it

A logical approach to serious kidney disorder is to do everything you possible can to lessen their load and to improve your nutrition. Your Nature Cure practitioner will be able to help you with this aspect of the changes you will need to make. The other important part of the picture is that your other blood-cleansing organs will need to be encouraged to accept their fair share of the load, indeed, probably more than their fair share for a while. Anything that encourages greater activity of your skin and more complete and vigorous breathing will all help to lessen the burden on your kidneys.

If you are suffering from kidney distress, then the citrus fruits, like lemons and grapefruit, are best avoided. Although oranges, mandarins and tangerines can be eaten as whole fruits – rather than squeezed as juice when it is all too easy to drink three oranges in one glassful – they should be eaten in moderation, and the fruit should be ripe and naturally sweet.

This contrasts strongly with the natural methods of assisting kidney function. Assuming, for the moment, that one of the original causes of your kidney overload was overeating animal proteins and this error has now being corrected, one of the most effective ways to benefit your system is bodily activity. Being up and about is infinitely more helpful to the kidneys than lying in bed.

An excellent way to assist your kidneys is the now familiar cold compress worn around the waist. Properly applied, and having produced the normal response of prolonged warmth and nervous relaxation, the compress aids the kidneys in two ways. It improves the circulation, enabling the blood to flow more freely and this means less physical strain on the tissues. Your backache might lessen and there can be a darkening of the colour of your urine. In simple terms, the work is being done more completely, with less exertion. More indirectly, the compress also encourages greater activity in skin and lungs. If you are not familiar with the application of the cold compress see the chapter 'Water and Nature Cure'. Manipulative treatment, in the form of massage can also be beneficial.

You can further help your kidneys to functioning more efficiently with the position you sleep in; this is because the position of the kidneys themselves is significant. If you sleep on your back, the kidneys are at a lower level than your bladder, so that there is a gradient and a potential for backpressure against which the kidneys must work to transfer the urine. When sleeping face down, gravity assists the flow from both kidneys, alternatively changing from one side to the other can give each kidney in turn a spell of easier working. These measures might seem small but can make the difference between waking with a clear head or feeling bleary and sluggish.

What can we help you with?

The Nature Cure treatment may be considered as consisting of three main parts.

Firstly, we try to discover what factors have produced your original overload, and as far as possible suggest corrections in such aspects as diet, posture and exercise. Secondly we encourage the other blood-cleansing organs to work more efficiently, so as to reduce the strain on your kidneys. This is sometimes called 'derivative' treatment, meaning that it is intended to direct the load away from the overworked area and on to tissues better able to cope. Thirdly, we attempt to remove all obstructions, physical, mental and emotional, that can so easily get in the way of proper nutrition reaching the kidneys and sustaining your whole person.

These categories of treatment in fact overlap considerably and, in addition, there is always the primary task of doing all possible to restore a normal balance and efficiency in your body's functions as a whole. One of our unique selling points is that we do not treat only the disease, we treat the whole person. Although it often seems as though we are only interested in what you are eating and drinking, in fact we are concerned with all aspects of your vital existence. The psychological and the somatic aspects will be investigated and your emotional state will be brought into the picture. It is pointless to give instruction only about dietetics to a person if their illness has been primarily caused by emotional distresses.

Healing activity

In any ordinary circumstances, reasonably vigorous exercise causes elimination of much more waste than it creates. We believe that you should remain as active as possible, within reason and your capabilities, as this assists your circulation as a whole and the activity of all your vital organs. Even if vigorous muscular activity is impossible, gentle regular movement should be attempted. Every so often some expert or another will suggest the use of the rocking-chair to assist the circulation, soothe the nerves, improve digestion or to achieve greater efficiency of respiration for those not in the best of health. My grandfather, in his book *The Heart*, published in 1937, mentioned the rocking chair as a valuable aid. Under the heading 'A Gentle Massage for the Vital Organs' he noted that 'The patient should spend as much time as possible during the day rocking gently in a rocking chair.' In 1937 orthodox reviewers expressed horror at the suggestion that the patient might do something active for themselves.

Liquids

The excessive intake of liquids of all kinds is possibly the biggest single feature in kidney disease. From spirits to coffee, lemonade to beer, black tea to beef tea, glucose and caffeine-laced energy drinks, juice drinks and bottled water we are all swallowing more and more liquid. We have already noted the damaging effects on the kidneys of certain ingredients in 'soft' drinks, but it should also be made clear that the absence of alcohol from a drink is no guarantee of its suitability or wholesomeness. There is another insidious chemical that can have far-reaching negative effects on your kidneys and some of you will be perfectly well aware of the cumulative and harmful effect of fluoride in drinking water, but it is worth reminding you of the susceptibility of the kidneys to damage from it. Kidney stones can contain up to 1,500 to 1,700 parts per million of this 'harmless' substance that is often added to many public water supply at 1ppm. When you are really thirsty probably the safest drink is plain mineral water in amounts adequate to slake any genuine thirst.

Points to remember

1. Get the bulk of your daily liquids form your food.

2. Eat a diet rich in fresh fruit, salads and vegetables. These should make up 70 per cent of your daily intake.

3. Stimulate your skin to greater activity to take some of the pressure off your kidneys. See the chapter 'Living Skin'.

4. Breathe deeply and exhale fully, get your ribcage moving and fully oxygenate your blood.

5. Take regular exercise and get your circulation flowing.

6. Avoid stressful situations and don't allow fear to dominate your thoughts.

7. Use a cold water waist compress – it is your kidneys' best friend.

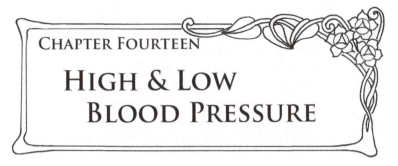

CHAPTER FOURTEEN

HIGH & LOW BLOOD PRESSURE

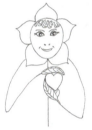

A WHILE AGO I overheard a conversation 'My doctor says I have blood pressure', the statement delivered in a gloomy tone of voice. This caused a little internal chuckle because if you didn't have blood pressure, you would no longer be alive. You might be one of the many unfortunate individuals who have been given a diagnosis and have been prescribed drugs to either raise or lower your blood pressure. But otherwise, have been given very little real explanation of what your diagnosis actually means.

As we have already observed in previous chapters, the state of your blood and its viscosity is affected by the health of your lungs, kidneys and skin. Your heart is the pump whose job is made easier, or harder, by the health or lowered level of activity of your other vital organs.

It is widely accepted that all blood pressure diagnoses must in some way indicate serious ill health, but the term really reflects a rather too broad description, often coupled with a lack of information. Blood pressure is essential to human life. Blood pressure means the force exerted by the blood on the vessels that contain it. Pressure is what causes the blood to flow along the vessels; the blood travels from wherever the pressure is high to wherever it is lower, in that respect behaving like any other fluid. The forces that drive blood flow are purely physical, and they depend on the differences in pressure in the various parts of the circuit.

There is no real meaning in the expression 'the blood pressure' as a fixed figure. Your blood is subject to many different pressures, according to where in your body it is located, at what phase of the pulse and, of course, the overall state of your body. Throughout life these factors produce a wide range of pressures, each of which is constantly varying. The highest pressure occurs within the powerfully muscular left side of the heart, when the contraction of the ventricle sends the blood out on its journey around the body. From this point, its pressure falls progressively until it has completed its circuit and arrives back in the thorax – as venous blood – to re-enter the heart.

Adequacy and effort

However, there are limits to the pressures that heart and vessels should be expected to accept if good health is to be maintained. Excessive pressures must impose excessive stresses, not only on your heart and blood vessels, but also on all the other tissues and organs in your body. Fortunately the range between adequacy and dangerous excess is wide under normal conditions. Throughout a reasonably healthy life the pressures of the blood vary considerably.

There is nothing alarming, or even unusual, about this. In perfectly healthy individuals, passing circumstances may call for exceptionally high pressures, although these should normally be of brief duration. Rapid alterations are not indicative of disorder; indeed, they may be confirmations of vigorous health. Only when high pressures remain after the need has passed do they suggest abnormality.

The heart is the hardest working organ in the body, ordinarily contracting about 60 to 75 times per minute. As each chamber of the heart relaxes, it is immediately refilled with blood, and this cycle is repeated, with amazingly few missed or imperfect beats, throughout your life. So long as you stay in good health, there is no strain; you remain quite unaware of the elegant balances and adjustments of your circulatory system.

Interpretation

It is the Nature Cure view that the idea of a fixed systolic pressure – or any other pressure – as an index of health is based on limited appreciation of cardiac and vascular function. The assertion that specific figures are characteristic of health or illness should be called into question. Yet this should not be taken as totally discounting the readings as valuable aids to the diagnosis and treatment of cardiac or circulatory disorders. So much depends upon the philosophy, training and interpretation of the individual practitioner, and at least as much on the recognition of overall circumstances when the readings are taken. It is for this reason that we may not only find our readings at variance with those obtained by another person, but can also come to quite different conclusions on the health and prospects of a patient even when the two sets of readings are broadly the same. This is but another way of saying that blood pressure and pulse readings have a significance that is far more subjective, and open to individual interpretation, than many specialist cardiologists would have us believe.

Normality and variation

Rapid fluctuations of blood pressure can be essential to health, and controls on blood pressure are exerted by living and adaptable mechanisms. If you are healthy, any change in pressure will occur only in response to a demand by some tissue, organ or system in your body. So, raised, or lowered, pressure is not in itself pathological if it is an action in response to some healthy irregularity in your body.

However, should the abnormally high pressures be sustained, other changes that could prove harmful can be induced. Some functions may be rendered less efficient by the excessive pressures, with progressively serious effects upon your general health. But this does not alter the fact that abnormally high pressure is primarily a consequence rather than a basic disorder. It is the effect, not the cause.

Influences

If you first draw a full, deep breath this will cause both systolic and diastolic pressures to immediately fall slightly. If you then exhale with similar vigour, this will cause a considerable increase in both pressures. With each action, your pulse rate is also influenced, speeding a little as the breath is drawn in and then slowing as the breath is driven out. Irritation, resentment and anger rapidly raise all pressures, whereas amusement and happy laughter can produce just as rapid a reduction.

To sit up, or stand, after lying down will cause the blood to gravitate toward abdomen and legs, with an immediate and considerable fall in pressures. In health, there is instant response and almost immediate compensation. Increased tone of the arterioles in the lower members restores pressure in the upper parts and, without any conscious effort or inconvenience; the entire bodily distribution is once more balanced. If your muscle tone is less than healthy you may experience a lack of blood to the upper parts of your body and a feeling of light-headedness.

Intelligence

If you seek to cure blood pressure disorders by medication, there is an almost total disregard of your body's own intelligence. Those with a true philosophical outlook recognise that what is regarded as 'effective' medication must also impose a totally artificial stress on the system. No matter how ingenious the method of administration or how accurately the dosage may be gauged, and it doesn't matter if it is of natural or chemical in origin, no drug has the ability to be aware of situations. A medication cannot know when it is necessary, when it should act and when it should be inert. It cannot detect the need of any vital organ at a particular time and weigh that need up against the requirements of the body as a whole. These things can only be adequately dealt with by your body's own somatic intelligence. And to the extent that any medication diminishes the promptness and accuracy of the 'computing' within that intelligence, it is a potential threat to your long term wellbeing and vital prospects.

When medication is prescribed there has generally been the assumption that there has been a breakdown in one or more of the systems in your body. More often than not we find that your body's somatic intelligence is rising with an amazing comprehension to address a collection of abysmal internal problems. There has come about, through a combination of unhealthy living habits and life's stresses and strains, an abnormal state of your organs and tissues. Therefore valiant efforts by your heart and vascular controls are required to sustain your vital processes. You might become aware that one day you can no longer run up stairs. You should recognise this as warning, but instead in dismay, you ask your doctor for something to bring back your stair climbing ability. Should the doctor oblige, then your body's intelligence will be overruled by a foreign agent, and you cease to be a self-regulating entity.

Anything that obstructs the free flow of blood from the heart, such as increased general nervous tension, prevents your heart muscle from contracting fully. Specifically, the left ventricle will not be emptied completely by the end of the contraction. So any residual blood within the ventricle is immediately added to by a full charge of fresh blood from the auricle above. This combined volume of blood distends the ventricle to a greater capacity than previous pulses. The muscle of the ventricle becomes more

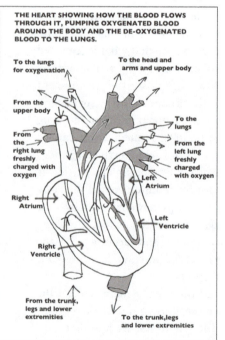

THE HEART SHOWING HOW THE BLOOD FLOWS THROUGH IT, PUMPING OXYGENATED BLOOD AROUND THE BODY AND THE DE-OXYGENATED BLOOD TO THE LUNGS.

To the lungs for oxygenation

To the head and arms and upper body

From the upper body

From the right lung freshly charged with oxygen

To the lungs

From the left lung freshly charged with oxygen

Left Atrium

Right Atrium

Left Ventricle

Right Ventricle

From the trunk, legs and lower extremities

To the trunk, legs and lower extremities

LIVE WELL. EAT WELL. BE WELL.

fully extended and, by the mechanism outlined above, exerts greater force on the blood. Usually within a few more pulses, the overall circulation is restored to its normal volume.

This automatic adjustment, due to the sensitivity of the heart's muscle fibres, happens within a few milliseconds. But don't underestimate the degree of compensation that might be made. It has been claimed that a healthy heart is capable of increasing its effort eightfold for short periods, all without prior warning, without delay and without distress. However, this situation cannot be allowed to run on indefinitely. All your vital organs have good reserves of ability, but the longer they are forced to run above normal levels the shorter the effective life you can expect of them. Other things being equal, a heart that has to work twice as hard cannot be expected to last as long as it might with more reasonable treatment.

Kidneys, adrenals and other glands

Sustained abnormal pressures can also have a devastating effect on your kidneys. In the condition known as nephritis, blood pressure figures can be dramatically high. It seems there is a kind of chain reaction at work, it starts with a generalised high blood pressure, produced by the factors discussed above, and in turn this affects the circulation of blood through your kidneys. A direct result of reduced blood-flow is diminished kidney activity, with diminished kidney activity there is a failure to excrete the very kind of wastes that contribute so markedly to your general hypertension. Greater obstruction is the result, and the difficulties of the kidneys are intensified.

The link between blood pressure, and its effect on blood vessels, and the adrenal glands – which sit on top of the kidneys

– is direct. In simplified terms the adrenals have two distinct regions. There is the inner, or medullary, portion, which has been described as 'the brain of the pressure system'. It consists of nerve-like matter interwoven with possibly the richest blood supply of any bodily organ. So with such an intimate relationship between the mat of tiny vessels and the nervous tissue, the medullary portion is able to respond instantly to changes in the composition of the blood, and to relate these to the overall nervous state of the system.

The outer layer of the adrenals, their cortex, is responsible for producing adrenalin of variable composition. Depending upon the proportions of its constituents, this has specific stimulant or depressant effects upon all the muscle types throughout the body. With the adrenals so closely related to the kidneys, when the kidneys are distressed the adrenals appear to suffer in sympathy; when the kidneys are functioning normally, the adrenals do likewise. Together, they may be beneficially influenced by some simple adjustments in your lifestyle, along with some other techniques in Nature Cure practice. Eating a more balanced diet, moderating your fluid intake, receiving some manipulative bodywork to release obstructing tensions in the region of the kidneys and related spinal nerve centres, and employing some simple external water applications, can all have a fairly direct beneficial effect upon your blood pressures.

Transporting wastes

If your diet and lifestyle are poor then your blood will almost constantly be carrying more than its fair share of potentially toxic matter, and this excess waste material can cause your blood to become thickened. The substances consist largely of acids of various kinds including hippuric, uric and beta-oxybutyric, and other assorted toxins. Because the acids tend to form the largest part we are liable to refer to the wastes collectively as 'acids', and this may give the incorrect impression that the bloodstream is itself made acid by their presence. In truth, the blood has the ability to absorb considerable quantities of waste acids without itself becoming acidic. However, the greater the acid content, the more viscous your blood becomes. This means that your heart has to work harder and when this occurs over a lengthy period, you might gradually become aware of various unpleasant sensations; chill, depression, lack of concentration and a general feeling of weariness. Often you will be tempted to use certain foods and 'near foods' to produce temporary relief from these distresses. This is where the popularity of tea and coffee becomes understandable. They apparently work in two ways, firstly by a direct stimulation, which releases additional energy from the body's vital reserves and, second, by a chemical effect upon the acidic burden of the bloodstream.

The initial boost, or 'upper', from the caffeine has the desired effect. But sadly in a short time this feeling of increased energy wears off, exhaustion or tiredness returns greater than before, and the 'downer' makes you feel worse. The sticky acids in the blood are to some extent precipitated by the active ingredients in the drinks. This means that your blood is in a more fluid state, but still containing crystals of acidic material. For a time, your blood will be circulating more freely, and for a limited period there is a feeling of greater wellbeing. But there is a problem with this solution; the crystalline acids have not been eliminated; they are still within your body. Some may be deposited in such tissues as joints, muscles or nerves, giving rise to the symptoms of arthritis, fibrositis or neuritis. But for the most part the strain falls on the walls of the blood vessels themselves. If this was only an occasional event then the walls could withstand the irritation, but the problems build up when the assault occurs several times per day and this is when chronic changes begin to occur. The arterial walls gradually become thickened and hardened; arterio-sclerosis has arrived.

Pulse rate

We have all taken our own pulses at one time or another and 72 beats per minute is the standard textbook number, but some say that anything between 60 and 100 beats per minute should be considered 'normal'. Your heart rate will change and adapt regularly as it adjusts to the activity you happen to be engaged in at the time. The rate will depend on what you are doing and how fit you are. The fitter you are the lower your resting rate should be and well trained athletes can have a resting rate as low as 50bpm for men and 54bpm for women in their mid-lives. It can be lower in younger age groups. Average rates are somewhere between 70 and 84 for late middle age, but whatever the figures, it is broadly true that the healthier you are the slower your rate will be when you are at rest. Orthodoxy has come a little way toward recognising this, by observing that well-trained athletes have resting pulse-rates 'considerably lower than normal'. We would say that even if you are non-competitive in your chosen exercise you are better off with a resting rate nearer to 60 than 72bpm.

Emotional distress

It has been said that 'thoughts are things', and they can certainly have undeniable effects on the behaviour of your heart and, of course, on the state of your blood vessels. Any kind of fear or anxiety will produce an immediate speeding up of your heart action and an increase of tension in the vessel-walls. This is due almost entirely to nervous responses, and both the pulse-rate and the pressure can fall back to normal in a relatively short time once the reason for your fear is removed. But when you are emotionally distressed over a long period of time the most constant factor appears to be resistance within the smallest arteries, the arterioles. For more explanation about the far reaching effects of stress see the chapter 'The Fear Factor'. Normally this resistance would cause the pulse rate to rise, but it is not possible for this extra effort to be continued indefinitely without risk of permanent damage.

When you get a fright adrenaline (epinephrine) is released into your bloodstream, this causes an increased volume of blood per minute to be pumped through your system, but once the danger is passed then your pulse rate falls back to a more or less normal figure. If the stress remains for a considerable time however, it can cause an alteration to your heart structure. The heart may take some considerable time to be effected by this mechanism, which is called compensation. A heart can also be referred to as 'enlarged'. If proper elasticity of the tissues is not maintained, the enlarged walls may yield and thus exert distorting strains upon the heart valves. 'Incompetence' is the danger here.

Towards recovery

It has often been stated that 'there are no apparent symptoms of high blood pressure'. Technically, that may be a correct observation, but it overlooks the many signs of stress throughout your body that may stem more or less directly from hypertension. It also overlooks the extraordinary efforts of your gastro-intestinal tract and your lungs to compensate for the shortcomings of your heart. Your skin may also act in a broadly self-sacrificing way, with pimples, pustules and boils, as well as more generalised rashes becoming apparent. These are all effective methods of helping to restore a workable state of blood-chemistry, even though they can be uncomfortable, potentially damaging and unattractive. Equally distressing though they may be, diarrhoea, vomiting or the production of copious catarrh from the lungs, might be some of the most effective ways for your body to maintain its vital functions.

Points to remember

1 Don't be frightened by a diagnosis of high or low blood pressure. It should be a spur to make healthy changes to your lifestyle.

2 Eat a balanced diet mainly made up of fresh fruit, salads and vegetables. Keep your extra fluid intake low.

3 Eat your meals in a calm, quiet environment or in a convivial one.

4 Take regular exercise that causes your heart rate to rise. This will bring oxygen into your system and the muscular exertions will assist your circulation.

5 Do some exercises that will help your abdominal tone. You will find some suggestions in the chapter on Posture and Movement.

6 Don't drink stimulants like tea, coffee and caffeinated soft drinks in an attempt to get more energy; you will just feel more tired later.

7 Avoid stressful situations and seek help with anxieties and worries that are keeping your blood pressure up.

8 If you are recovering from 'heart problems' be prepared to take some extra rest if you are tired, until you are feeling better.

LIVE WELL. EAT WELL. BE WELL.

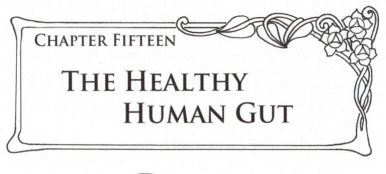

CHAPTER FIFTEEN

THE HEALTHY HUMAN GUT

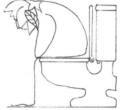

THE PHYSIOLOGY OF digestion will be broadly covered in the chapter 'What To Eat For Health' and most people already have a basic knowledge of the anatomy of the alimentary tract from school biology lessons. What we will be looking at is the Nature Cure way to achieve a happier digestive system and how to gain a better understanding of our ailments.

All of us suffer from constipation at one time or another during our lifetimes, often without actually realising it. No matter how good your diet is, if you have an emotional crisis, or your work situation is making you over-anxious, then there will be some disruption to the normal functioning of your gut.

My grandfather, through his work at Dr Henry Lindlahr's[1] sanitarium in Illinois, started to understand more fully the importance of a healthy digestive system. He set about collecting as much information about the gut from as many different sources as he could. The result was what he called his 'sixty-piece jigsaw'. These pieces he eventually assembled into what was probably his most ambitious piece of writing, *Constipation and Our Civilisation*, a book based on over a quarter-century of professional experience. It was first published in 1943.

The origins of this short chapter date back to his book, the value of which was quickly recognised as a fundamental contribution to the understanding of health by many of his contemporaries. Sir Albert Howard, an English botanist, an organic farming pioneer, and a principal figure in the early organic movement, called it 'a remarkable book that must be read'.

There is not enough room in this book to list all 60 pieces of information my grandfather deemed essential, and some have since been modified but the ten listed below still ring true today.

A ten-piece jigsaw puzzle

1   It is natural for the bowel to contain discarded and decaying food waste; also small amounts of broken-down and discarded body constituents. Therefore the bowel must be designed to resist absorption – or re-absorption – of such toxic substances.

2   What is inside the bowel is outside of the body. Your finger in the hole of a doughnut is not in the substance of the doughnut.

3   Although only an elongated 'hole in the doughnut', the human alimentary tract is designed to retard the passage of food material at its later and most decomposed stages. This tells us something about the kinds of food for which it is

intended – as do many other features of the structure of our gut.

4   Dryness of faecal matter acts as a stimulus for the production of mucus fluids. To inject water is to remove that stimulus, and so results in a still more constipated state. Any natural function of the body that is not used tends to atrophy. The more you do for your body, the less it will do for itself.

5   The sick human is too often encouraged to eat, to 'keep up his strength'. The sick dog does not eat. Most wild animals go through annual spells of living with little or no food. Civilised man and animals in zoos rarely do. Civilised man and zoo animals often tend towards unhealthiness.

6   Body weight is not necessarily a good indicator of health. Being overweight or underweight does not necessarily mean you are unhealthy, but equally being the ideal weight does not guarantee good health either. Disease can be present in any body size.

7   The real danger in constipation is that toxic matter may seep from the bowel into the bloodstream. This is most likely to occur when: i) a poor diet produces abnormal concentrations of toxins in the bowel ii) the bowel wall is rendered less resistant by medication iii) the bowel wall is thinned by over-distension or iv) flow through the bowel walls is increased by injected water.

8   To eat decaying food in small quantities is not dangerous to robust health. To eat perfectly sound food in quantities too great for the digestive juices to cope with, and for the body to absorb without distress, is to invite putrescence in the bowel. A large mass of toxic material is a potential danger.

9 Most people's problem is that they want to eat, drink and do things that are not good for them. They also hope to be healthy while doing so. If you stop doing the things that are making you ill, you start to become healthier. If you don't stop the unhelpful habits, ultimately you have 'incurable disease'.

10 Constipation is but one aspect of a general disorder. To cure constipation, every aspect of health should be looked at. To seek and apply a remedy for a single symptom makes a real recovery unlikely.

Fasting and enemas

Even though you might not feel particularly unwell, some of the symptoms you feel when constipated will point towards you having toxic wastes stored in your tissues to a greater or lesser extent. This soured state of your tissues including your bloodstream, may be described in a variety of ways: acidosis (an abnormal increase in blood acidity), toxaemia (a condition characterised by the presence of bacterial toxins in the blood) or autointoxication (poisoning by a toxin formed within the body itself). 'Health or death begins in the colon', is an observation first ascribed to Dr Bernard Jensen[2] and in almost every case constipation is part of the picture. This might sound strange, but, constipation is a much-misunderstood term and what follows is an attempt to explain its true significance.

In his student days in the United States, my grandfather witnessed the treatment of seriously ill patients with a variety of mono-diets, such as milk or fruit, with different periods of fasting, plus daily enemas. In most cases the patients appeared to be restored to enthusiastic health with great speed and certainty. But unhappily those rapid recoveries did not stay cured, and he found confirmation of his own early experience, as a desperately ill young man, that temporary relief is all too often a trap for the unwary. In addition to this there was a limit to what any given patient could stand in prolonged fasting. A patient's own estimate of their condition can be totally unreliable, in fact, enthusiasm can be the first sign of emotional instability, so that it is essential for there to be professional supervision of any fast longer than a few days. The individual can be quite convinced that they are making steady improvement, when all the objective signs are of a serious deterioration of their condition.

Causes

There is any amount of written and spoken information about constipation, yet it remains one of the most commom – and possibly the most medicated – conditions. This failure arises because almost no attention is paid to original causes. Instead, there is an enormous market for medicines, remedies and appliances offered to deal with the problem, ranging from ethical prescriptions, through patent medicines, herbal mixtures, 'health' foods, and enemas of all kinds, to the everlasting advice to 'drink plenty of fluids'. The latter advice is given in a vain attempt to flush out the bowels.

Less waste

However, it is not necessarily abnormal for your body to need a bowel evacuation only once per day, or two days, or even a week. If you are eating the absolute minimum necessary to sustain health, and thus encouraging the gut to use almost everything, there will be little bulk of waste. If, in addition, there is no abnormal discharge of catarrh or other body-wastes into the intestine, there may not be enough faecal matter to justify opening the bowel more often. To quote Horace Fletcher[3] who earned himself the nickname 'The Great Masticator' by arguing that each mouthful of food should be chewed at least 32 times:

> Following the ingestion of a lessened quantity of food and its better assimilation, there is less waste. The lower bowel is not the reservoir it formerly was. So haemorrhoids cease from troubling and constipation cannot exist.

Quick fix

It is only human nature to look for an instant cure, and even when you truly believe that you are seeking an alternative method of treatment, too often these largely are no more than variants of symptom suppression. Once you have lost faith in laxatives you might believe that you have found a fundamentally different approach in colonic irrigation: in truth both methods have the same aim – to induce a bowel movement by increasing the liquid content of the bowel and by causing irritation of the bowel walls. Neither method can have a truly beneficial effect on the basic distress because neither of them does anything to remove the predisposing stresses on your system or to improve your eating habits. Put simply, these remedies do not remove the causes of your condition.

Sufferers of chronic or regular bouts of constipation often take too little exercise, and also tend regularly to overeat, they also drink too much liquid. In addition to cups of tea and coffee, glasses of water are drunk throughout their waking hours and sometimes when they wake up in the night as well. This excessive water intake is often intended to 'cure constipation', and is resorted to as a substitute for medication or enemas. Sadly, as a remedy for the problem it is just as detrimental to the system and ultimately just as ineffective.

Water addiction

But surely there is no harm in the habit of water drinking, apart from the high price that the environment pays with the amount of plastic waste that results from so many of us discarding our plastic bottles. Where is the harm in drinking water in quantity? Surely what the body doesn't use will just get passed as extra urine, won't it? Well, it's not that simple, and we have looked at the extra work your kidneys are obliged to do if your liquid intake is out of proportion to your true need. For those of us living in the Northern Hemisphere, when we are well nourished, eating a balanced diet full of fresh fruit, salads and vegetables, very little extra fluid is needed to keep us fully hydrated.

Sudden collapse

When the kidneys fail to keep up with unfair demands on them fluid retention can be the result. This is most readily recognised by the skin taking on a lasting imprint of tight underwear. This condition is known as surface oedema, and it basically represents so much undischarged urine. It is often accompanied by the typically sallow complexion of uraemia and sometimes with a fullness of the figure that can be easily mistaken for robustness. Such individuals are liable to collapse suddenly, with pneumonia or comparable signs of vital failure, 'while in perfect health'. Just as with the mistaken belief that 'the strongest and healthiest' are most prone to certain other forms of disease, the truth is often something quite different.

The fatal mistake lies in misunderstanding the signs: if you are a truly healthy person you will not die from sudden disease. The spectacular diseases that are said to attack victims without warning are almost always of slow growth and development. For those trained to recognise the signs, there are plenty of warnings. So, if we stop overeating and stop overdrinking then 'sudden' emergency diseases will virtually disappear. As we explored in the chapters 'The Living Skin' and 'The Fear Factor', watery tissues have very little resistance to any physical or emotional strains. It is within such tissues that 'sudden diseases' occur.

Drinking between meals

Apart from the total quantity of water we drink each day there is the important consideration of when it is drunk. If all our food were truly natural and wholesome, the question of drinking with meals would rarely arise, and drinking between meals would be minimal. However, for newcomers to a Nature Cure way of life it can be distinctly uncomfortable to have nothing at all to drink with a meal, even if a drink with food is not truly normal. Wild animals only visit the watering hole once a day and tend not to drink if their mouths are full of food. However, real dryness should be at least eased with a moderate amount of liquid, though you will find that as you wean yourself off the highly spiced foods and on to more natural and subtle tastes your thirst will reduce accordingly. Largely, drinking with meals is habit rather than need. How often do we see people take a huge mouthful of sandwich and immediately 'wash it down' with a gulp of tea, with barely a chew to start the starch digestion in the mouth?

Once your meal is finished, and the digestive processes have got under way, the stomach should have no further food or drink until the next mealtime. It is important to allow the digestive processes to be carried out without interruption. Those engaged in vigorous activity may find this difficult, as thirst may well be genuinely greater than in a less active person. Much of what we think of as thirst is largely imagined and habitual, but if you do find it is really intense it may indicate an abnormal and irritable state of stomach and intestines. Your thirst may not be so much a bodily need for fluid as a call from the digestive tract for dilution of irritants. This dilution gives only temporary relief; the proper course is to recognise and avoid the foodstuffs that cause the abnormal thirst and the ideal is to avoid any large amounts of liquid between meals.

Miss a meal so you can enjoy the next one more

If you feel really thirsty, then we suggest that you take only simple liquids at the next mealtime, on the principle that avoiding further solid food should allow the gastric surfaces to recover from the irritation that the previous meal has caused. Try just having a glass of water or a small amount of a slightly diluted real fruit juice (Not a 'juice drink' which is generally full of synthetic sweeteners). Don't go for a huge mug of tea or coffee (even the decaffeinated varieties) and alcoholic drinks are not suitable either. Yet, how often do you have a cup of coffee or a mug of tea instead of food when short of time? Just remember Dr John Tilden's 'Rule No.1', 'Never eat unless comfortable in mind and body from the previous mealtime.'[4]

He went on to explain, 'If this rule is carried out whenever discomfort occurs, it means missing only one meal. But if discomfort is allowed to continue, without regard to this simple formula, the rest required may run to several days before the digestion becomes comfortable again.' This latter advice is really useful, and does mean that by simply skipping one meal you can get back to sensible eating and lose the discomfort of indigestion so much sooner. Emotional eaters have a habit of stuffing their feelings back down their throats with food and while this might seem like a comforting thing to do at the time, taking a short, brisk walk in the fresh air can offer a much better outcome. If your situation will not allow you to do this, some quiet deep breathing can be helpful.

As explained above, in the temperate climates of the Northern Hemisphere, a diet containing plenty of raw salads, raw or simply cooked vegetables and fresh fruit should provide almost all the fluid required for efficient bodily function. We recommend that 60–70 per cent of your diet should be made up of these constituents. We also suggest that by eating a vegetarian diet, and avoiding flesh-foods, that there is less potential for the build up of irritant and toxic waste in your system, and so far less call for dilution to prevent distress.

Cold, hot or spicy

Your stomach and its contents must reach blood heat before digestive action becomes truly effective. If cold water or iced foods are eaten in any quantity, these can seriously delay digestion. Cold water should therefore be taken in sips, each warmed in the mouth before swallowing, and similarly foods like ice cream should be eaten slowly and in moderation. Note the 'brain freeze' reaction when you eat cold foods too quickly or in too great a quantity.

Hot drinks can be damaging too. When we take anything too hot into our mouths we tend to hold on to it or try to swallow it as quickly as possible when we should really spit it out immediately. Early training in politeness stops us from doing this in company, and instead we swallow the mouthful. There might be immediate relief from the pain in your mouth, but the damage internally can be severe. Although being scalded, the walls of the stomach cannot signal the fact, and the injured surfaces can become sites for potential ulcers or other degenerative changes. In this way, gastric disorders develop 'without cause or warning'. Worse still are the results of a research project published by the British Medical Journal in March 2009.[5] This project involved tea drinkers in northern Iran where their teas are traditionally drunk at a high temperature. It was found that the hotter the tea was when being swallowed, the greater the risk of the individual developing oesophageal cancer.

And it is not only hot-in-temperature foods that burn the linings of the gut. Highly spiced foods such as chilli peppers can cause burns too. Try scooping out the seeds from a hot chilli with your bare hands and the capsaicin oil in them will burn your skin. If you have started to become de-sensitised to that burning sensation then take it as a warning to cut them out of your food list. Chilli pepper extract is a chief active ingredient in pepper spray, which is commonly used for self-defence. Just because other people seem to add chilli to everything these days it doesn't mean that it is a good thing. No other animal causes themselves that level of pain with no real nutritional value to offset it.

Breaking habits

Generally when your health is depressed it dulls your normal, self-protective reactions. However, not everyone believes just how powerfully self-destructive forces can operate. It all seems so contrary to what we believe about ourselves, and about our natural instincts. Some of us are only too happy to continue our bad eating habits, we tell ourselves that it is okay because we can offset it by the exercise we take every day, however, it is our finding that the greatest resistance is to giving up the very habit that is most destructive. The man killing himself with tobacco may cheerfully give up coffee. Someone addicted to his or her ten cups of tea every day can do without the occasional alcoholic drink. It is as if we do actually recognise, at a subconscious level, where our problems lie; the person with a damaging habit tries to avoid any reference to it. So often in practice we have found patients trying to guide our enquiries away from any potentially damaging habits. This is why we find it is so important to treat the whole person, not just the symptoms being talked about.

So, where does ill health come from?

Free advice is always suspect, and never more so than in matters of health. Unfortunately, the converse is not always true; paid-for advice is often coloured by some self-interest of the seller. In such a complicated situation, we ought to be able to fall back on our instincts, but we have already seen that instincts can become confused. So where can you look for reliable guidance? Perhaps five points offered, with typically uncompromising bluntness, by my grandfather so many years ago may provide a sense of direction:

1   Disease never arises without a cause.
2   Anyone who offers a short cut to health ignoring cause is a quack, no matter how he may be acclaimed.
3   Belief in cure without removal of cause is probably the most dangerous fallacy of the present day.
4   Only your own inherent vital forces can cure you, and while the causes of disease remain these vital forces cannot succeed.

LIVE WELL. EAT WELL. BE WELL.

5   Although many ailing people seek out and appear to enjoy humbug, Nature is not impressed.

We believe that the above is still true today. You will also see from the above why Nature Cure practitioners refuse to endorse or approve whatever the current trendy treatment happens to be. Too many of them are merely variations on an orthodox approach, selling herbal substances that are substitutes for the pharmaceutical equivalent, both claiming to cure this or that ailment. Some of these remedies work by suggestion and may indeed produce a change in symptom but they nearly all ignore causes and concentrate upon quick end results; the suppression of symptoms. Symptoms can be powerful signposts to the actual cause of your disease or distress, but avoiding getting down to the roots of your problems is a highly profitable business. Pretty packaging and an almost instant relief from those annoying symptoms, however transient, is so much more attractive than having to accept that fundamental changes to your lifestyle will need to be made to achieve truly robust good health.

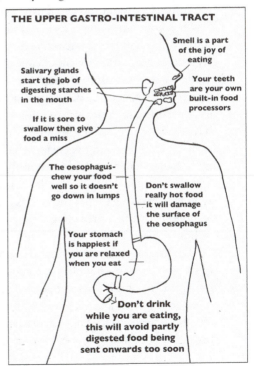

THE UPPER GASTRO-INTESTINAL TRACT

Smell is a part of the joy of eating

Salivary glands start the job of digesting starches in the mouth

Your teeth are your own built-in food processors

If it is sore to swallow then give food a miss

The oesophagus- chew your food well so it doesn't go down in lumps

Don't swallow really hot food it will damage the surface of the oesophagus

Your stomach is happiest if you are relaxed when you eat

Don't drink while you are eating, this will avoid partly digested food being sent onwards too soon

Chronic causes

It would be much more helpful if we could make a more honest assessment of how lives are blighted by familiar yet ultimately destructive habits and customs. The fact that most serious illness results from either an excessive absorption of toxic matter from the gut, or a failure to rid the tissues of toxins, or a combination of both, is rarely recognised. That all acute infectious diseases are generally constitutional and heavily reliant on a pre-existing condition is not often appreciated. It doesn't matter how it is described, the search is still to find that magic bullet that can kill the invader without too-obviously also killing the invaded.

Such common signs as a coated tongue and unpleasant breath (often called halitosis, a term coined by a mouthwash manufacturer who needed a market for the chemical solution that was originally made to sterilise surgical instruments) are indicative of serious intestinal disorder. Yet these warning signs are so often accepted as normal and provide rather useful selling points for synthetically-flavoured, medicated toothpastes. Those same companies and their clever advertising agencies which successfully persuade the mass-consumer to eat denatured rubbish masquerading as 'wholesome' food, are happy to make further income from boosting symptom-masking preparations. It is the familiar case of one abuse leading to another, providing multiplied profit for the exploiters of human nature. It would be funny if it weren't so tragic.

The gradualness of physical deterioration over the years, due to daily errors and human slips and strays, work insidiously on our constitutions. It doesn't matter if they are everyday household remedies or socially acceptable stimulants, tea, coffee, alcohol, etc, the symptom-masking agents produce an inevitable level of breakdown. Apparently without any dramatic preamble, you are

LIVE WELL. EAT WELL. BE WELL.

suddenly struck down with a heart attack, kidney disease, diabetes, stroke or cancer. And it cannot be the denatured foodstuff, the aspirin, the antacid, the tobacco, the tea, the coffee, the sleeping pill or whatever, which is responsible, because you have taken these for years and this has never happened before. In the present context, laxatives are also high on the list of potential dangers. They are both symptom-maskers and causes of chronic irritation to your vital tissues.

All the stimulants, which so many of us are accustomed to drinking, and many of us have come to depend upon, begin by producing a natural revulsion. But persistence, aided by the expressed or tacit approval of already-addicted friends and family, leads to what we euphemistically call 'tolerance'. This is in truth the stage at which your body has become so depressed that it no longer bothers to react to the abuse; you are no longer repelled by bitter taste, too-hot foods, acrid fumes or uncomfortable responses.

In my grandfather's words:

From birth, civilised man's toleration to habit is built up in an ascending spiral, and all habits inhibit awareness. If the first effect is stimulation, the inevitable reaction is enervation. Enervated (weakened) organs and nerves are less under control and use up much more vitality. Hence the deadly tiredness so often complained of by those who are deteriorating into an 'incurable' condition. There is no easy way out for such individuals. Stimulants must be given up until vitality returns, and even then it may take a considerable time before a useful reserve of nervous energy can be built up.

If recognised in the earlier stages, and stimulating habits are given up before serious indications show, health may return quickly.

In all this, it should not be overlooked that one of the commonest stimulants is an excess of food. This is especially the case where refined products make up the bulk, but even natural sugars and proteins can act as powerful stimulants when taken in quantity.

An added aspect of trying to regain and maintain good health is the level of background environmental pollution that we all have to live with. Unnatural man-made chemical pollutants are so insidious that it is almost impossible to fully protect yourself from them. All you can do is eliminate them from your home and the immediate environment within your control. Even something as apparently innocuous as washing up liquid, if not properly rinsed off your crockery and cutlery, can cause long-term digestive upset.

Masked constipation

Those of us who habitually overeat, or who have lost the ability

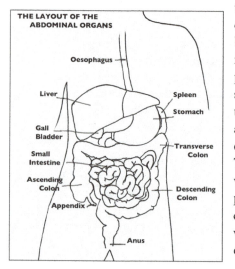

THE LAYOUT OF THE ABDOMINAL ORGANS

Oesophagus

Liver

Spleen

Stomach

Gall Bladder

Transverse Colon

Small Intestine

Ascending Colon

Descending Colon

Appendix

Anus

to extract vital nutrients efficiently, may have regular, daily bowel movements, yet suffer from constipation. This can persist for years, with no symptom more severe than tiredness and frequent headaches. The sufferer is seldom ill enough to need to stay in bed. The abnormally large residues within the digestive tract over pack the colon, which is never completely emptied. In other words, what should have been discharged on Wednesday does not appear until Friday or Saturday, or even until the following week, but because there is a daily evacuation the situation is rarely recognised for what it is.

This induces, in fact, the worst feature of constipation; an excessive flow of toxic substances from bowel to bloodstream. The body must rid itself of this toxic embarrassment somehow, and skin rashes or catarrh are commonly the result. Such escape routes may enable the body to function well enough, but if something – such as suppressive treatment – causes obstruction of the supplementary eliminative effort, then more serious developments are likely to occur. These may range from chronic anxiety and mental irritability to such crippling disorders as severe rheumatism and cardiac incompetence.

Give your guts a rest

Emotional troubles or upsets interfere both with restful sleep and with efficient digestion. At times of anxiety or severe stress, give your gut a rest from food. This will not leave you undernourished, it will, on the contrary, release some energy for repair and restorative activity. It should also help to redevelop a true hunger instinct and this is a precious asset that so few of us possess these days. As explored often in previous chapters, change is difficult and challenging for us, and imbalances in our diet can lead us to resent new ideas. There is such a close relationships between the food we eat and the way we behave that faulty nutrition can all too easily lead to bad judgements and flawed decisions.

Wild animals, in their natural environment, make few feeding mistakes. Domesticated animals can be persuaded to accept unsuitable foods, but even they are not easily coaxed to eat when in pain or if they are ill, stressed or over-excited.

To fast or to eat

It is important here to stress the difference between having a short rest from food, routine weekly 24 hour fasts and pure fasting. What has been described above is a short rest from food in response to a particular condition. In a weekly 24 hour fast you would take nothing but water from, for instance, lunchtime one day until lunchtime the next but in pure fasting nothing whatsoever, except water, is taken, which means that your body has to operate within the limits of energy and materials already stored in its tissues and organs. In very few cases is there any serious shortage of potential energy – in the form of fat and of sugars – but there are almost always serious deficiencies in vitamins and organised minerals. It is the lack of these vital elements that can cause anything from severe to complete obstruction to the processes of healing and repair. That is, the patient may, for a few days, benefit from lifting the load of digestion, but thereafter little of lasting benefit happens.

However, it is one of the primary teachings of Nature Cure that anyone who is going through an acute illness has little or no need to eat much, or indeed to eat anything. Your body almost certainly has adequate reserves to carry through the healing crisis to completion. If there is a raised temperature, the ban on food is even more essential; a feverish body has more than adequate reserves, and adding fuel can only prolong the fever. The advantages of avoiding food during acute illness are so obvious that some are encouraged to take this one step further, if abstaining from food is good when you are undergoing a healing crisis then why not keep it up after the acute phase is over? They regard a fast as the universal treatment for all ailments – even those attributable to prolonged malnutrition. In simplified terms, we see a fast as an opportunity for an over-driven body to catch up with its repairs and maintenance work, unimpeded by the considerable demands of digestive activity. Therefore, by implication, the system must possess adequate supplies of materials and potential energy before a fast can be fully exploited positively.

If you are truly undernourished then your body will not be able to make effective use of a fast, even though the diminished availability of energy may produce a dramatic cessation of some of your more unpleasant symptoms. In some extreme cases we see a fast as being as suppressive and destructive as any medication. If you are new to Nature Cure then any attempts at fasting for more than 24 hours should be supervised.

With the above caveat, let us look at some of the positive benefits that may follow abstention from food. Most Nature Cure practitioners would probably use the term 'long fast' for a pure fast of more than a week, but mostly we favour short fasts repeated at intervals. Freed from fear, an ordinary person, without preparation, can probably go for several days without any food and with only water to drink and suffer no harm. The older established religions nearly all involve fasting as an obligatory observance. What abstention may produce in religious credit is at least equalled by the physiological benefits. It is altogether wholesome to run down the store cupboards occasionally before restocking with fresh. A fair proportion of our long-term adherents make a regular practice of having one fast day per week. For those who were perhaps faced with a grave prognosis tens of years ago, such 'sacrifice' seems a small effort in return for continuing an active survival. It does seem, in many cases, to make all the difference between keeping going, without any major breakdown, and suffering frequent off-days and relapses. However, it is important that the one-day-a week faster should not think that this can somehow take the place of reasonable daily routines, it is an additional observance.

Koumiss and lettuce

In Kingston's earlier days, a large number of new patients were considered to be hopeless and had come to us as 'incurable'. For them, it was essential to introduce some healthy bacteria into their unhealthy guts. The Clinics's preferred method gave their bodies the easiest possible access to beneficial flora; they were given nothing more to eat or drink than small portions of Koumiss (soured raw, unpasteurised organic milk) and a few leaves of lettuce, three or four times per day. There will be more discussion of milk in the chapter 'What To Eat For Health'.

With a limited supply of fresh vegetable and of bacterially active soured milk, these two together supply vitally-significant amounts of vitamins and minerals, they enable the body to release further supplies from 'locked' stores and from undigested food substances already present. The total bulk of koumiss and lettuce is small, far too little for the nutrient content alone to account for the impressive increase in energy and self-reparative efforts. It is the combination of koumiss and lettuces' 'vitalising' elements, the existing and newly released reserves and the freedom from incessant and fatiguing digestive turmoil that together produce seemingly miraculous results in desperate cases.

Koumiss and Lettuce is not specific as a treatment; it is no more than a shorthand to describe the provision of an activating diet to meet the patient's needs at a given time of difficulty, while avoiding as far as possible any digestive overload. 'The least necessary' is the guiding principle.

We have all been firmly led to believe that 'germs cause disease' and too many of us find it hard to believe that all higher forms of life depend directly upon myriads of germs. When the advertisement tells us proudly that a particular disinfectant 'Kills 99 per cent of all known germs', it omits to mention that 99 per cent of all known germs form a vital and active part in supporting life on Earth. We as a species would be quite quickly extinguished by sterility – an absence of germs in our environment – as we are well adapted to existing in close relationship with the 99 per cent of beneficent microorganisms. The calculation is that a healthy human gastrointestinal tract could be home to some 100 Trillion microorganisms weighing in at nearly 3kg of gut flora.

Less is more

It is over 400 years since an Italian nobleman – Luigi Cornaro (1467–1566)[6] wrote his 'Discourses on a Sober and Temperate Life', Luigi was a sick and weak man at the age of 40 with a very poor prognosis, but by changing his diet and exercising some considerable self-discipline he enjoyed another 58 years of excellent health. He gave the world this epitomised advice:

> He who would eat much must eat little; for eating little lengthens a man's life, and by living longer he may eat more.

He lived to 98, active, alert and cheerful to the last.

References

1 Dr Lindlahr, Henry (1862–1924), The father of modern Nature Cure.
2 Jensen, Bernard D.C., PhD, The father of Holistic Health.
3 Kuhne, Louis (1835–1901) Naturopath and Hydrotherapist.
4 Tilden, Dr John Henry (1851–1940).
5 Ref: *British Medical Journal* in March 2009 Research BMJ 2009; 338 doi: http://dx.doi.org/10.1136/bmj.b929 (Published 27 March 2009).
6 Cornaro, Luigi (1467–1566) 'Discourses on a Sober and Temperate Life'.

POINTS TO REMEMBER FOR A HEALTHY GUT

1   Eat wholesome foods in moderate amounts.

2   Avoid excessive liquid intake – any type of liquid, including water – and don't drink with food at mealtimes.

3   Avoid laxatives and enemas, they only treat your symptoms and are not a cure. They can become habit forming and undermine your body's natural processes.

4   Be careful about the types of foods you eat together in combination at meal times, some mixtures can be difficult for your body to digest properly.

5   For further information about food combinations, amounts and recipes see the chapter 'What To Eat For Health'.

6   Eat starches, sugars, proteins and fats in moderation. If you eat 60–70 per cent fresh fruit, salads and vegetables in a balanced diet you can't go far wrong.

7   Eat fats and proteins that are as simple and unprocessed as possible. We all need some fats and proteins to keep a healthy physiology.

8   Avoid processed and denatured starchy and sugary foods – and non-foods.

9   Don't overcook your food; eat raw as much as possible.

10 There could be a spinal or other anatomical displacements causing your discomfort, have your frame checked by a qualified naturopath or osteopath. Out-of-place bones can affect your nervous system, your circulation and your digestion.

11 Excessive work, and the resultant weariness, can compromise the efficient working of your digestive system.

12 Don't eat when you are upset or worried, emotional stresses can play havoc with your digestion.

13 Avoid taking any sleeping pills or sedative drugs, they don't just make you sleepy.

LIVE WELL. EAT WELL. BE WELL.

14 Keep your intake of tea, coffee or alcohol to a minimum – or stop them altogether.

15 Don't smoke – it's not just your lungs that are affected, every cell of your body is too.

16 Avoid the use of vitamin pills, eating a sensible honest balanced diet will provide you with all the vitamins, minerals and trace elements that your body needs in a far easier to use form.

17 Avoid any habit or occupation that causes you to consume large amounts of nervous energy. A tired body cannot be expected to make the best use of food.

18 If you are feeling down or are suffering from depression seek some professional help, but also try to be careful about your choice of foods and take as much exercise in the fresh air as possible.

19 Try to do some inverted exercises each day, even if it's just for a few minutes. Good tone in your abdominal muscles helps your guts function better.

20 Try to have your cold-water Squat Splash each morning, preferably following your inverted exercises. For more information about hydrotherapy for home use see the chapter 'Water and Nature Cure'.

21 Avoid taking painkillers, they do not cure anything, they only mask the symptoms; try using a cold waist compress.

22 Try to avoid taking blood pressure regulating or allergy drugs; these and other medications will interrupt your normal digestive processes.

23 Avoid antacids, stop drinking while you are eating and make sure you eat slowly and chew your food well. Don't swallow hot drinks until they have cooled sufficiently.

24 Fear in all its forms will cause your digestive system distress, try to address your fears and don't eat if you are agitated or upset. See the chapter 'The Fear Factor' for more information.

PART THREE

The Nature Cure approach to diet and preferred food types has changed little since 1912. But so much else has. Nobody could have foreseen the proliferation of agri-businesses so heavily dependent on fossil fuels and chemical inputs that occurred during the last century. No one could have imagined the rise of the multi-national food giants with their universal production of highly processed foods and near-foods. This "progress' seeming to move hand-in-hand with a sad, but avoidable, increase in chronic illnesses. Throughout the same period our aims and ideals held fast. We have always championed wholefoods and unprocessed food and recommended a varied Organic, plant-based diet. This section will help you to make food choices that are not only healthy for you and but kinder to our shared planet too.

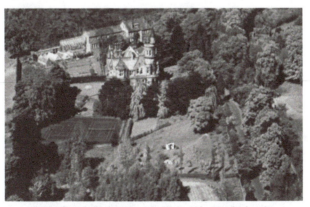

An aerial view of the Kingston Clinic and grounds showing the large organic kitchen garden and glasshouses where we grew salad greens and vegetables all year round.

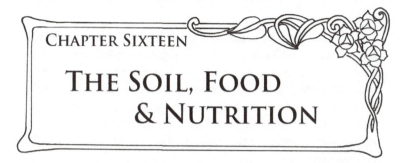

CHAPTER SIXTEEN

THE SOIL, FOOD & NUTRITION

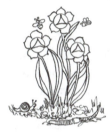

THE KINGSTON TRAINED Nature Cure practitioners have always linked the health of your environment with the state of your health. Particular emphasis has been put on the quality of the soil, principally because your body gets the building blocks it needs to rebuild or maintain health from the food that you eat. It is a simple correlation that if the food you eat is highly processed, full of trans fats and fructose from corn syrup and, at the same time, lacking in organised vitamins and minerals, then you cannot expect your body to be truly healthy. If you want proof, it can be found from one of the biggest unplanned randomised trials of all time illustrating the importance of a good diet, just look at the difference in health between those eating a reasonably balanced diet and those who eat predominately 'junk' food.

It is sad that high input, chemical dependent farming is now considered to be 'conventional'. It might be good for big agri-businesses, but it isn't good for our long-term health, the health of our children, the health of animals or the health of the soil. To a Nature Cure follower conventional should mean organic, sustainable, free of toxic chemicals and working with the laws of return with respect for the land, the farm, wild animals and the environment.

The Soil Association and many grassroots groups have helped to highlight our unsustainable dependence on fossil fuels that is favoured by the current conventional farming system. Our government and the EU back high profit and quick return intensive farming. Radical changes are needed to the way that our food is produced and to the way that our farm animals are reared and kept. Vegetable crops are hauled long distances by road to centralised packing stations, often hundreds of miles from the fields where they were grown, and then transported, often back over the very same roads to supermarkets and eventually to consumers. Good prices in the supermarkets mean producers being pushed to the limits on costs. Mixed production family farms struggle to compete with the huge agri-business farms specialising in arable, dairy or meat production.

It is impossible to divorce the health of the soil from the health of the food that is grown on it, or from the health of the individual, animal or human, eating that food. Ideally foods should be sourced as locally as possible, eaten as unprocessed as possible, mostly eaten raw or conservatively cooked and grown in our own window boxes, gardens or allotments.

When buying fruit and vegetables from any source it is worth being on your guard; you might be eating a veritable rainbow of different coloured fruits and vegetables all uniform in shape, colour and size. But you might also inadvertently be taking in doses of pesticide, insecticide or fungicide when you eat them. At least with organically grown food you substantially reduce that possibility. And if you still think conventional farming is the only way to feed the world, recent research has found that some 30 per cent of non-organic bread in the UK is contaminated by glyphosate, a widely used weed killer. Hardly the stuff for building a healthy population.

Circularity

Nutrition is a basic biological necessity and is required for all living things. In its simplest form it is a flow of nutrients and energy between organisms and the environment. This flow is cyclical and is totally interconnected, from minute soil organisms to plants, to animals and us and back, eventually, to the soil.

Although it might not seem immediately apparent, soil is the obvious starting point when talking about food quality. Most of the foods that we eat rely on soil at some point in their lifetime. Of course there are exceptions, for instance, with hydroponic and aquaponic systems but these rely heavily on – often artificial – fertilisers rather than healthy soils for growth. The condition and treatment of our soils will have a knock-on effect on health all the way up the food chain. The fertility of a soil is essential for healthy crop growth but for organic farmers and gardeners – including permaculturalists and bio-dynamic growers – that is only one aspect of many. For those growing by any of the less 'conventional' methods, biodiversity is key to a healthy system.

What do we mean by 'soil'?

Here is Lady Eve Balfour's[1] description:

> Soil is a universal storehouse covering most of the habitable land mass of the world where nature lays up supplies of its essential building blocks, its activity is biological, chemical and physical. The biological function of soil includes the processes whereby the raw materials contained in minerals and in dead and decaying plant and animal materials are made available for new plant growth.

The abundance of organisms in soil is staggering, with some 22 tons of fungi and bacteria in an acre of good quality soil, and whilst it is true that not all bacteria are helpful to the grower, a greater number are essential to plant growth. A wide range of fungi exist in fertile soil, many associated with the breakdown of dead plant materials, recycling a whole range of essential chemicals into the soil.

Mycorrhizal fungi play a vital role in the uptake of nitrogen; the fungi form an association with the fine roots of a huge range of plants. This is a symbiotic relationship, with the fungi receiving sustenance from the roots of the plants and repaying this by assisting their host in the uptake of nitrogen.

Earthworms

Not all soil organisms are of a microscopic scale. The earthworm has a hugely beneficial effect, moving significant volumes of soil up from deeper levels. Through their daily ingestion and movement of soil, earthworms bring accumulations of nitrogen, phosphates and potash to the surface via their casts, these deposits on the surface are weathered back in and taken up by the shallower roots of plants. The earthworms also aerate the soil by burrowing

LIVE WELL. EAT WELL. BE WELL.

deeply and they enable oxygen to reach the lower roots. Charles Darwin[2] studied earthworms and investigated the changes they could make to an area of soil through their daily movements:

> There is good evidence that on each acre of land, which is sufficiently damp and not too sandy, gravelly or rocky for worms to inhabit, a weight of more than ten tons of earth annually passes through their bodies and is brought to the surface.[2]

There can be as many as eight million earthworms in one acre of healthy soil, but in some areas their numbers have been reduced by up to 30 per cent by the inadvertent introduction of the New Zealand flatworm. These rather unpleasant creatures live off earthworms and have few natural predators in this country. The flatworms have been in the UK since 1965, arriving on imported garden plants. The long-term effect on the health of the soil from the loss of earthworms is still being investigated, but as some earthworms form burrows that assist with drainage there is some evidence that the lack of earthworms could be contributing to flooding. Look out for molehills; where there are molehills there are earthworms and no flatworms.

Manure

The application of composted materials or well-rotted manure to the soil is a vital part of the 'law of return', or putting as much in as we take out. This helps to ensure good soil health – and good heart – and goes a long way towards true sustainability. Conversely, the effects of chemical high intensive input agriculture on a piece of land can be very damaging, yet may take many years to show. It will depend in a great part on the health and structure of the soil in the first place. A field that has been part of a rotation system with roots, cereals, stock and grass leys being followed in a four or five year cycle will have a level of fertility built up in the soil. Intensive production relying on chemical inputs alone will be boosted by the inherent health of the soil for the first few years, as well as the nutrients derived from the dead bodies of the earthworms, but the lack of genuine input will eventually become apparent. As the crops start to show distress the problem will inevitably be addressed with further applications of chemicals. These denatured soils are far more vulnerable to erosion and flood damage than those with good rotational use, good structure and good heart.

Artificial fertilisers

I vividly recall a friend talking about putting manure onto her horses' pasture – the 'manure' she referred to was a bag of ammonium nitrate in small white pellet form... how our perception of what the word 'manure' actually means has changed.

The real and genuine nutritional value of crops grown by the intensive method also has to be questioned. New or novel strains are bred to cope with chemical cocktails and this changes the fundamental makeup of the plants. Modern bread wheats have a far greater gluten content than older strains, newer ones allowing manufacturers to make fluffier white bread. Common sense would lead us to make a link between changes to the wheat and the growing number of individuals suffering from gluten intolerance.

There are many old varieties of wheat, and other cereals, which are no longer used in food production to any great extent, and this is partly due to the costs of registering seeds to meet EU regulations. This is a great shame because a pioneering experiment at the Long

LIVE WELL. EAT WELL. BE WELL.

Ashton Research Station near Bristol[3] found that many modern crop varieties are poorly suited to low-input, organic farming systems. Most modern crops are grown purely for high yield. Any disease-resistance or standing ability is given a far lower priority by the breeders. Therefore farmers using these modern varieties have to apply a mind-boggling selection of chemical sprays to overcome their weaknesses.

The government argues that we need to grow intensively to feed the hungry population, they give financial support to farmers to grow crops intensively and the agro-chemical industries back them to the hilt and bank the profits. So the comforting picture of a farmer in touch and in tune with the soil that supports him and his family and is providing good honest food crops is mostly a thing of the past. The truth is likely to be a contractor, working for an absentee landlord, cocooned in a fantastically expensive tractor fitted with computers and satellite-navigation equipment that can tell them exactly how much seed they have drilled or how much of any particular chemical they have spread.

Sick land – sick people?

In his excellent book *The Killing of the Countryside*, author Graham Harvey[4] explores the current relationship between the land and those who work it, and finds that:

> Everywhere on these islands rich and beautiful habitats have been ploughed, bulldozed and sprayed out of existence, not as a result of need, but in response to farm subsidies.

Although the gleaming brightly lit supermarket with its endless aisles of packaged and processed food may seem a world away from the farmer's field, the choices that the busy, often harassed, shopper makes influence directly the vitality, health and bio-diversity of our countryside and the food that we eat. There is a direct link between the health of our soils and the profits of the supermarkets. As the one gets poorer, the other grows richer:

> A farming system that produces a sick countryside will
> eventually produces a sick population.[4]

Simple wholesome diets equals good health

Weston Price[5] in his major work *Nutrition and Physical Degeneration* illustrates many instances of healthy populations of indigenous people who lived good and productive lives on very simple fare. The mountain people in Switzerland, the plains Indians of America, even the older crofters in the western isles of Scotland all worked the land, grew their own grains or greens, raised a few animals and ate their own dairy foods, fish and a little meat. They were fine specimens, strong and muscular from physical work with excellent teeth. Within a generation of being introduced to white flour, white bread and tinned foods they had suffered from dental caries and had started to lose their health; tuberculosis being the most common physical disease in Scotland. When they took the last residents off St Kilda, the small group of islands some 40 miles west of the Outer Hebrides in 1920, to resettle them in 'better housing' on the mainland, there were three women over 85 in the population.

Genetically Modified Organisms

Genetically Modified Organisms are out there whether we like it or not; they have been introduced into the food chain, often through the back door in animal feeds and often with the blessing of the powers that be, even though the UK is ostensibly a GM free zone:

LIVE WELL. EAT WELL. BE WELL.

In global terms the use of GM crops has increased steadily since the first commercial plantings in North America in the late 1990s. By 2014 about 18 million farmers in 28 countries were growing GM crops on 181 million hectares, which is 13 per cent of the world's arable land.[5]

In theory, there are currently no GM (GMO) crops being grown commercially in the UK. Imported GM foods, however, especially soya, are being used in animal feed, and to a lesser extent in some human food products and vegetables. This means that they are in our food chain and effectively 'the genie is out of the bottle'.

There is the further issue of a tiny handful of huge multinational companies having control over the grain that subsistence farmers in the third world can sow, claiming to have the copyright for that grain in perpetuity. This is clearly neither ethical nor fair. Vandana Shiva[6] has highlighted the numbers of third world farmers who are committing suicide because they can no longer afford to buy the seed annually. In the past farmers could save seeds from the previous year's crop for future planting, but this is not permitted with GM seeds as it is an infringement of copyright. Vandana describes this as 'food totalitarianism' and in August 2014 she addressed a gathering at a seed fair in Florence:

> There are two trends; one: a trend of diversity, democracy, freedom, joy, culture; people celebrating their lives. And the other: monocultures, deadness. Everyone depressed. Everyone on Prozac. More and more young people unemployed.

One of the stated advantages of GM crops is that they are herbicide resistant so they can be sprayed with high levels of glyphosate based weed killers and still survive, but recently glyphosate, a weed killer that is in universal use in parks, gardens and farms all over the world, has been shown to be somewhat less benign than first thought. Glyphosate was the weed killer that was 'safe' for pets and children and became magically neutralised when it hit the soil. It is still the top selling weed killer and the one favoured by the manufacturers of genetically modified organisms, however, it is now being implicated in the death of human cells. And if it kills human cells it will also kill animal cells. Several different research projects have shown that one of glyphosate based Roundup's supposedly inert ingredients actually amplifies the toxic effect on contact with human cells, even at concentrations much more diluted than those used on many farms and GM crops, and that it is this combination that makes it particularly damaging to embryonic, placental and umbilical cord cells. So in the end the only truly safe weed killers are a Dutch hoe, some elbow grease and a bit of mulching. Although you can use boiling water to kill weeds too.

Pesticides

Chemical residues in our foods have wide ranging health implications and have been linked to decreased human – and almost certainly also animal – fertility in males and are suspected to be a major cause of food allergy and intolerance. There has been a massive rise in the number of people suffering from food related illnesses in the last few decades and this cannot be purely coincidental. Of course, the causes must be multifactorial, but the over processing and poisoning of our basic foodstuffs with repeated chemical applications has to be among them. Recently the routine use of neonicotinoids to treat seeds has been highlighted because of the tragic decline in our wild bee and honeybee populations. The seeds of rapeseed are coated to stop them from being eaten in the ground, but because it is a systemic weed killer the substances persists even in the flowers at levels that have badly affected our bees. This sorry tale should give us all pause for thought.

We are encouraged by the Government to eat Five-a-Day. But recent testing of basic fruit and vegetables grown by conventional methods has found significant amounts of pesticide residues in pre-packed salads, apples, strawberries, pears and carrots. The government guidelines[7] consider these to be at 'safe' levels using their 'Maximum Residues Levels' yardstick. However, Dr Clare Butler Ellis of the Pesticide Action Network said:

> The pesticide Residues Committee almost always finds 'no cause for concern' with these levels of pesticides, but we think the public is right to be concerned and to try to so something about it.[8]

'Ordinary' (white) bread, farmed fish, 'speciality' beans, okra, pulses and chilli peppers all showed significant levels of pesticide residues. The organic products tested from the same categories showed no residues whatsoever.

Pesticide residues have been implicated in decreased fertility in humans and are suspected to be a major cause of food allergy and intolerance. That there has been a massive rise in the number of people suffering from food related illnesses in the last few decades cannot be denied. There are undoubtedly many – probably inter-related – reasons for this, but the processing and poisoning of our basic foodstuffs is undoubtedly one of them. It is hardly surprising that there is little appetite for research in this field; big business has nothing to gain and a lot to lose from the probable findings.

So it is worth paying more for organic food

When we consume conventionally grown, high input fruit and vegetables, we are supporting the big agro-chemical industries and also perpetuating our dependence on fossil fuels. Non-organic growing also requires the liberal use of artificial fertilisers and these do not return anything to the soil. The Nature Cure preference is to eat organic, locally produced food, as in tune with the seasons as possible. This cuts down on the amount of fuels used for the transporting of goods and helps us to live in a more natural, holistic and sustainable way. It also means that we are eating foods that our bodies are adapted to cope with.

Unless it is contra-indicated by your current state of health, the Nature Cure diet will include a modest amount of dairy products as part of its overall balance, but the emphasis is on the word modest. As usual the recommendation is to buy organic, as organic farms do not use antibiotics as growth promoters, they have a lower stocking density of animals and the expectation is for lower yields of milk and eggs. The animals are allowed much more freedom to roam and are expected to gain the bulk of their feeding from natural sources and grass pasture.

Another good reason to eat only organic animal products, and then in moderation, is that if you choose conventionally farmed foods, you are likely to be getting a daily dose of antibiotics. And these antibiotics, used as growth promoters, might just be linked to our current obesity epidemic, if groundbreaking work by Martin Blaser[9] is correct. He, and his team of scientists at New York University, questioned why antibiotics made farm animals bigger and fatter and carried out research to find the answers using mice. The team produced evidence showing that the female mice given a sub therapeutic antibiotic treatment in their water laid

LIVE WELL. EAT WELL. BE WELL.

down more fat over the same time period than the control mice on pure water. They were surprised to find that within a few weeks bone growth was also affected and this too was considerably greater. The results were not unique to one type of antibiotic, but present across all the drugs tested. From the findings during his extensive research Martin Blaser suggested that the low doses of antibiotics present in animal derived foods are having a major influence on the size and weight of the people who eat them. This finding could go some way towards offering another explanation for the massive rise in obesity in recent years. And yet another good reason to eat organic – especially dairy produce and meat.

Do we need meat to get enough protein?

The short answer is no, we can get more than enough protein from organic dairy and vegetable sources. But the issue of whether or not to eat meat isn't really the point, it is more about the issue of eating *too much* meat and too much protein in general. For many people, meat is the main part of a meal, they feel cheated without it and greenery is there only as a slightly begrudged garnish. A shift in emphasis to the meat being the garnish and the greenery being the main bulk of the meal is required to obtain a better balance. Out of preference most Nature Cure followers eat a plant-based diet, and for some body types this is really the best option, but equally some people do eat a little meat and fish.

Even those of us who rely on nuts or pulses for our proteins should be mindful of where they come from and the air miles that they can clock up. Although hazelnuts and walnuts will grow in this country they are rarely grown here on any commercial scale. It is possible to buy cashew and hazelnuts from fair trade or organic sources and this means that they are at least ethical.

According to BBC *Wildlife* Magazine:

> Cashews from India and Mozambique, and supplied by farmers
> who are shareholders in their own businesses... tend not to be
> associated with large-scale habitat destruction. In India they
> are planted as windbreaks and to provide shelter; they also
> help to stabilise sand dunes and protect the land... Lentils are
> grown in Turkey, which is one of the three main producers.
> Their cultivation is not associated with any habitat loss – indeed
> WWF Turkey says they help to enrich the soil and do not require
> significant pesticide use.[10]

So it is possible to find pulses and nuts that will not kill the planet,
and being dried goods they can travel by sea rather than air. But
they should really only be eaten in moderation and as part of a
balanced vegetable and fruit based diet.

Superfoods

There are myriad articles in the popular press about 'Superfoods'
and how this one or that one will miraculously change your life
for the better. Rest assured there are no Superfoods; health comes
from a balanced diet, not one magic vegetable or fruit in particular.
Constituents of food do not work in isolation, we need a range
and a balance of the right foods to get our quota of what we call
organised minerals. These organised or micro-minerals are also
referred to as trace elements and include iron, cobalt, chromium,
copper, iodine, manganese, selenium, zinc and molybdenum. Also
included are the essential vitamins, which are required as nutrients
in very small amounts by your body. And you can add to this list
the phytochemicals – chemicals from plants – these are compounds
that occur naturally in living plants. Some are responsible for

colour, some for taste and others for smell; think of the deep purple of beetroot, the taste of strawberries and the smell of garlic.

However, research has shown that the vitamin content of food is declining and comparisons between two extensive reports published in 1953 and 2001 illustrate this. Spinach saw a 45 per cent drop in vitamin c, beets were the same and broccoli dropped across the board with a staggering 60 per cent drop in vitamin v. The report also showed drops in vitamin a, calcium, potassium and magnesium. Corn (maize) has been a staple of many populations in the Americas, and this vegetable has seen a drop of calcium content by some 78 per cent.[11]

What do we need to eat?

The lists of foods we need to eat to obtain our full quota of vitamins, minerals and trace elements is relatively short, and its length in recent times has been influenced more by availability than necessity. If you look at any list of vitamins and minerals, the catch all term 'green leafy vegetables' appears very regularly, as do oats, legumes, carrots, brown rice, wholemeal bread, eggs and some dairy. This sounds remarkably like the range of foods identified by Maisie Stevens in *The Good Scots Diet – What Happened To It?*[11]

Stevens looks at The Statistical Account of 1790 which found the people of Fortingall in Perthshire to be 'in general long lived, many between 80 and 90'. Their diet according to her research was: potatoes, oatmeal, kale, turnips, barley, butter, cheese, milk and ale. She describes it as plain but wholesome and perhaps a little monotonous. But it had all the ingredients needed to build healthy, active, long-lived people.

The joy of growing your own

One aspect of food that cannot be ignored is the importance of growing your own. The excitement of sowing a tiny seed in compost and waiting for the first shoots to show, the enjoyment of planting out the growing seedlings, tending them and eventually harvesting the mature plant. If you produce it yourself you know exactly where your food originated and what went into it and the freshness is unequalled. The backache from digging, weeding and turning the compost heap can also serve as a reminder of exactly where food comes from and just how much energy goes into producing it.

Coming back briefly to the subject of those ubiquitous green leafy vegetables, their importance cannot be stressed enough and they include everything from lettuce to brassicas to herbs to leaf beets and spinach (the latter is best picked a few hours before eating to allow the oxalic acid levels to drop). We can grow lettuce and leaf beets in pots and sprout seeds, so even if we don't have access to a garden we can still grow greens for ourselves.

Food versus nutrition

So, the health of the soil is vital and it supports much more than just the food that we eat. Our food and what we eat is more than simply nutrition and food adds up to more than its component parts. The nourishment we derive from food can be as much about the people we eat with, where we eat or when we eat as it is about what we eat.

There are endless books written about food, nutrition, calories and diets. You can read all about food, junk foods, organic foods, wholesome foods, and foods that can all be counted in calories.

They tell you what every morsel can do for you, good or bad. There is no doubt that it is very important to eat a 'good' diet to maintain a reasonable level of health. With incidences of diabetes, heart disease and obesity increasing, even orthodox health practitioners now have to acknowledge that there is a strong correlation between what their patients eat and their state of health. And yet few, if any, of these books on food seems to be interested in the complete sustenance of the individual, or on the quality of sustaining the whole person; they are mainly concerned with nutrition on a building blocks level. Of course we need air and water too – we can survive for three minutes without air, three days without water and three weeks without food – but how long without contact and interaction with other living beings? Three months? Three years?

Food alone does not nourish us, and I am not talking about the current problems caused by the empty calories of modern convenience foods. You can eat the best organic, well balanced diet with every one of the 2,000 calories brimming with nutrition and goodness but you can still be left with a hunger that simply cannot be satisfied. No matter what you eat, that hunger remains. No cake, no bun, not even the best chocolate will fill the hole. The emptiness or hunger experienced by so many of us when our close relationships no longer nourish us will not be satiated no matter how many treats we ram down our throats. And that lack of emotional nutrition can make our health fail faster than a poorly balanced diet.

The emotional aspects of life can have a devastating effect on even the best diet. As illustrated in the chapters on 'Your Health and Your Emotions' and 'The Fear Factor' emotional turmoil will activate the stress response from our sympathetic nervous system.

Through the endocrine system the fight or flight response is instigated and partially – or fully – shuts down the digestive system. Prolonged emotional distress can seriously compromise the health of even the most careful of eaters.

The phrases 'starved of affection', 'a feast for the eyes', or even 'drinking in the views' have been adopted into common parlance for a very good reason. The world around us nourishes us too. This aspect of our health tends to be overshadowed by the subject that exercises the Nature Cure adherent more than any – food – and I would be the last one to decry the place of a well-balanced enjoyable selection of wholesome foodstuffs in a healthy person's life, but it is just one essential part.

The definition of nutrition

If you look up the word 'Nutrition' in a dictionary and then in a Thesaurus you will find 'sustenance' as one of the synonyms. If you then go back to the OED you will find 'the quality of being sustained' under 'sustenance'.

There is no doubt a healthy, well balanced, preferably local and ethically produced diet is vital to good long-term health; but it can also become an unhealthy obsession. One glass of wine does not destroy your liver or one bar of chocolate turn you into a diabetic. Eating the perfect diet does not automatically assure that you become a happy, balanced or healthy person.

How miserable we feel when we are weakened and lethargic from lack of exercise and how good we feel when we reach the top of the mountain and look back over the miles we have climbed and drink in the views. Even more amazing is how little fuel we need to achieve that climb; exercise of the right sort is an appetite suppressant.

Food, how we grow it, prepare it, and eat it is a huge part of the human way of life. Just take a look at the TV schedules or wander along the food section of your nearest large bookstore, and you will find endless advice on ways to cook and eat your meals. Feasts and festivals are all reasons for celebrating with food, and the sharing of food has huge significance. The family meal, a much-neglected event in many modern households, should be a pivotal part of everyday life for children of all ages. To sit down and eat with your partner, parents, or parent, and siblings should be a time for catching up with the news of the day and reinforcing family bonds. The downside is that the table can often be a battle ground too, as it is the one time in the day when all the family is together and actually has time to talk.

Creativity

As a final note it is worth mentioning the importance of creativity to the nourishment of the soul and body. Many of us have unsatisfying jobs and too little time for any form of creativity, but you don't need to be a great painter, singer or musician to be creative. Just enjoy making something, bake a loaf of bread, cook a simple meal, knit a hat or grow some flowers.

Nourishment, the act of being sustained, comes in many forms.

References

1   Balfour, Lady Eve, *The Living Soil*. Universe Books.
2   Darwin, Charles, *The Formation of Vegetable Mould*. John Murray 1904.
3   Ashton Research Centre, Bristol. Closed in 2003.
4   Harvey, Graham, *The Killing of the Countryside*. Jonathan Cape. Pages 6, 105 and 140.

5 Price DDS, Weston. Nutrition and Physical Degeneration.

6 Shiva, Vandana. Speech at Seed Fair in Venice August 2014.

7 Figures from Government Pesticide Residues Committee Report 2006.

8 Pesticides Residues Committee.

9 Blaser, Martin MD. Missing Microbes. Oneworld Publications. 2014.

10 Source: BBC *Wildlife* Magazine. March 2010.

11 Soil and Health.org Website 2015.

12 Stevens, Maizie. *The Good Scots Diet – What Happened To It?* Aberdeen University Press.

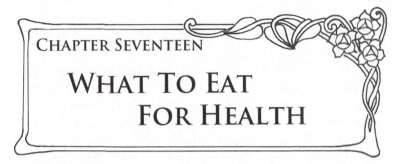

CHAPTER SEVENTEEN

WHAT TO EAT FOR HEALTH

The practicalities of sensible eating – also known as food reform

AS EXPLORED IN the last chapter, and throughout this book, one of the foundation stones of Nature Cure is the strong and undeniable connection between what you eat, and your state of health; your health is intimately linked with your nutrition. Although the importance of this aspect of healthy living has been understood for years, interest in the subject tends to wax and wane with the latest findings. The numbers of people taking their diet seriously does not seem to have grown as widely as might have been expected with the advent of widely spread nutrition information and diet trends. The burgeoning of health food shops around 30 or 40 years ago did not lead to a huge number of them on high street, although they are now a well-established minority feature in our food shopping landscape.

However, at this point it should be made clear that there is no such things as a 'health food' or a 'super food', but there certainly are healthy foods. There are all sorts of claims made about 'health foods' and 'super foods' but health cannot be obtained from jars, packets or cartons or even from one specific type of food. Health is not a commodity that can be bought or sold, it is a state of being. Foods need to be wholesome, eaten in compatible combinations and include a predominance of fresh fruit and vegetables to be truly nourishing and healthy.

The science of nutrition is very complicated and includes physiology, chemical reactions and physical activity, and these in turn are all affected by the emotional state. However, the basic art of eating for health is fairly simple if some basic guidelines are followed. All living organisms absorb food, break it down and then reassemble the component parts into their own substance. When your food supplies all the necessary ingredients it is nutritious, and a good balance and sufficient volume is best, but a constant over-supply of nutritious food does not necessarily produce better health. Too much food, like too much of anything, will congest your system, while too little will reduce its efficiency.

By-products of the internal combustion of the foods that we eat are wastes and have to be removed. Food must be made up of constituents that your cleansing organs: the skin, bowels, liver, kidneys and lungs, can easily make use of, and materials that are needed to nourish the body's tissue but will not overload the blood. Therefore we need to ensure that we eat a good balance of what we call the cleansing foods. These are salads, vegetables and fruits and they are water rich; real living foods. These should ideally make up 65–70 per cent of your food intake.

Functions of food

These may be simply described as:

1   Supplying energy and heat.
2   Building and repairing bodily tissues.
3   Providing specific substances such as vitamins, minerals and trace elements.

There is little doubt that the art of genuinely eating sensibly has largely been lost in the western world. The demands of our modern society have put pressure on working women and men and it is just too easy to pick up a ready meal or carry out on the way home rather than spend time preparing fresh food. But when you simplify your eating habits it becomes remarkably easy. There are endless magazine articles, and internet sites, devoted to the topic of healthy eating, one month it is this wonder food that will change your life and then next month it's another. The government exhorts us to eat our five-a-day, but since such foods as tinned spaghetti qualify on the grounds of containing tomato sauce there is every reason to suspect that it is big business' health that will be improved by this scheme, not yours.

But what is nutrition? It is certainly more than just the food on our plates, and the food itself is more than a collection of vitamins, minerals, trace elements and fibre. Food should be a vibrant living health-giving balance of taste, texture and calorific value. If we live on denatured, processed foods, eating more and more calories in the form of crisps, sugary drinks and chocolate bars, we will end up suffering from a form of malnutrition. This may sound counterintuitive, but sadly it is the case because the food we are eating does not contain the right nutrients. Our appetite is controlled by the pituitary gland, this is a small gland at the base of the skull and it is constantly seeking satiety through finding the vitamins, minerals and trace elements in our food that the body needs to function properly. If the food we eat does not have the nourishment that we need the pituitary will keep sending messages to the brain claiming that it is still 'hungry' because it had not been fed *properly*.

Wholesome and honest

So we need to eat good honest wholesome food, avoiding processed junk foods, but how do we know what is good for us and why? Freshness and nutrient content vary between different vegetables, even between vegetables of the same type, depending on the methods of production. Unless the vegetable is home grown or organically produced then you will almost certainly have to accept a level of pesticide, herbicide and insecticide residues on your plate. Most vegetables and salads on the supermarket shelves are put through a chlorine bath to ensure they stay fresh for as long as possible, and although this might be good for the producers and packers it is not quite so good for you because there is no real safe limit for organochlorides (recently some producers have started to label their vegetables and salads as being washed in spring water, and this is at least a better choice). So although you might be doing your very best to eat 'healthily' you could still be ingesting some unpleasant and unwanted chemicals. Research has shown that organic produce has a higher level of vitamins and minerals than the same types grown conventionally. (See the Chapter 'The Soil, Food, Nutrition and Nourishment'). This is a topic regularly debated in the popular press, but the one thing you can be assured of is that poisonous residues in organic vegetables are less than 30 per cent of the levels found in conventionally grown foods.

In addition to the above, Washington State University[1] carried out a meta-analysis of literature and research on the comparative micronutrient levels in organically grown vegetables and fruit versus the same types of produces conventionally grown. The results were published in 2014 in the British Journal of Nutrition. Eighteen scientists compared the data and discovered that not only were pesticide residues far lower or non-existent in the organically grown foods, heavy metal traces were also much lower. Better still, micro-nutrient levels were considerably higher. In 2002 the University of Missouri also identified lower nitrate levels, 50 per cent more vitamin c and higher levels of essential micronutrients in organically grown fruit and vegetables.

It is a shame that many people think that good, healthy food is beyond their pocket, as it doesn't need to be. Eat less, eat simple and grow some of your own – even if it's in a window box or a seed sprouter – and eating a reasonably healthy and balanced diet need not cost you more than using conventional or convenience foods. In fact, eating simply and healthily can be cheaper; try joining a food co-op who can buy dried foods in bulk, buy root vegetables that keep well rather than greens, and grow your own greens in pots, window boxes or in a seed sprouter. Most households throw out between £400 and £500 worth of food every year. That's a lot of organic fruit and vegetables that could have been bought and eaten.

There are so many reasons to choose organic, not least the fact that you are reducing your exposure to potentially damaging substances. The Nature Cure view is that acute illness flourishes where there is a pre-existing condition, and this condition can come about for many reasons. Adding external poisons to any toxins that are already accumulating in your tissues is to invite an extraordinary cleansing effort by your body. Sadly even the best foods tend to have some levels of contaminants in them these days. Add to this mix your general lifestyle, your emotional state and your stress levels, all of which have an effect on your overall health and digestive efficiency. Once you're aware of that list it is all too easy to see how toxic residues can start to build up despite your best efforts. When the accumulation is too great it will be a signal for the body to start a dynamic, and sometimes uncomfortable, cleansing process, the Healing Crisis. We liken this to a spring cleaning of your home; an extra-ordinary clearing out of accumulated wastes. This is an effort by your body to rid your tissues of their excess burden and is fundamentally a health-restoring measure.

The nature cure way with meals

Food was always a favourite topic at the Friday Questions sessions at the Kingston Clinic in Edinburgh. My father generally chaired these events and he was often assailed with versions of the same question, which is worse, tea or coffee? Is beer worse for you than tea? How much lettuce should I eat to get healthy? How much cheese is bad for me? In an attempt to answer some of the issues that surround food, what follows are some simple guidelines and the reasons for those recommendations.

Balanced nutrition is vital to good health, but it is not always necessary to balance your diet on a day-to-day basis. The proportions of different foods can be adequately maintained over the course of a week or maybe even over a month. Historically, when freshly picked or caught foods formed a larger part of the diet; the year was the natural period over which to achieve the balance. So if you choose to become a one, two or three meals a day eater you can still enjoy all the good foods available, simply give priority to those of different types at consecutive meals. Obviously the more meals you eat per day, the greater freedom you will have to choose from the different food groups. The reasons for avoiding certain food combinations will be discussed later.

LIVE WELL. EAT WELL. BE WELL.

Don't obsess over every mouthful

It is easy to give too much attention to every mouthful of food and often this can be counterproductive to achieving good health. It is important not to become over concerned about mixing this food with that, and to start fretting about what their combination might do to your digestion. Anxiety will adversely affect your digestion. So, it should be made clear that although some serious illnesses or disease types might demand strict demarcation between the different groups of foodstuffs, if your health is good and your digestion normal then there is a remarkably large amount of leeway around what can and cannot be eaten in combination. More often it is the amount of food being consumed that causes the distress to the system – rather than the type of food.

If you are the sort of person for whom food has been a bit of a battlefield, with regular dieting and weight loss followed by weight gain, then it might take some time for your natural appetite to re-establish. You might view salads as the punishment for putting on weight, rather than as a wonderfully satisfying and nourishing meal with an almost infinite variety of textures and colours.

Food addictions

It might strike you as an exaggeration, but it has been one of our findings that once someone has got into the habit of relying on a predominantly starchy and sugary diet we would effectively consider this to be an addiction or a dependency. Of course, we all need to eat, but some of us build up an excessive reliance on a disproportionate amount of one food or another. It is this type of habit that can so easily put our diets seriously out of balance. The food manufacturers are not stupid and they know that our craving is more likely to be for refined flour goods, sugary confections and salty snacks; the supermarket shelves are full of them. It's not only humans who fall into this trap, other primates kept in captivity will, given the choice, often eat the junk food first. That aside, it has been our long-term clinical observations that have confirmed our view about the term 'addiction', and the damage that seemingly innocent habits can do in the long term. You might have cravings, for instance, for refined starchy food and without your excessive daily intake of bread you start to feel miserable; when you get your 'fix' you are temporarily satisfied, but this feel-good situation is followed a short time later by a renewed feeling of despondency and a lack of energy. Sometimes, you can find other foods that can give you some temporary relief, and this might be considered to be a 'remedy' for the craving. However, they really do nothing to improve the essential situation; transferring an addiction is much the same as altering a symptom – only the outward appearance is changed, the fundamental distress remains.

To cook or not to cook...

Ideally, if you are in reasonably good health, in order to get the greatest benefit from the foods you eat they should be consumed raw or very simply cooked. Again, seek advice. If your health is poor and your gut efficiency is compromised you may find that the tough fibre of raw vegetables is difficult for you to break down. Care is needed when cooking because over-cooking vegetables will run the risk of losing too much of the valuable nutrients contained by their cell walls. The heat applied causes breakdown of the cellular fibre, and whilst this makes the food more tender and can also enhance the flavour, there will also be a loss of essential nutrients. The advantage of cooking is that it does make the remaining nutrients more available. Heat accelerates the progressive deterioration of the foodstuff, and as the nutrients are made more available by the action of heat they are also degraded, partly by the heat itself, and partly by the intermingling of different constituents within the food. Therefore, truly good healthy cooking means finding the briefest and lowest application of heat that will make the food enjoyable and palatable. While cooking means more deterioration, mixing too many different ingredients can confuse the digestive juices, hence our preferred avoidance of over-seasoned or too herb-rich dishes. By this definition many of the great cooks, who make dishes using complicated, multi-stage cooking – so beloved of the cookery shows – are sadly, dietetically speaking, the worst. By the time you have baked, steamed, fried and boiled all the different components there is a huge loss of essential nutrients. Perhaps we should follow Ghandi's example and only have five different foods on our plate at any time.

In general, the shortest and simplest method of cooking is the best. If you cannot chew well then juicing or fine grating is one route to getting a good selection of living foods. If you want to cook, then steaming or boiling vegetables in as little water as possible for as short a time as necessary should retain the greatest amount of micronutrients. There is also some research that suggests vegetables retain more of their vitamin and mineral goodness when steamed rather than boiled. Whichever method you choose the least possible cooking time and the least exposure to heat is the best way to retain the nutritional value of your food. It is worth considering the fact that vegetables have their highest nutrient content immediately after they are picked, and that the smaller they are the faster they lose their nutritional value. It is not only heat that can start to leach goodness, light and air can also begin the process. Ideally we should eat our vegetables and salads straight from the garden just after we have picked them and out of preference we should eat vegetables in their skins, unless they are too tough and unpalatable. However, it has been found that frozen peas can have a higher accessible level of vitamin C than garden fresh ones.

You may have been in the habit, for various reasons, of cooking your food at moderate-temperature over long periods of time. This has been shown to cause the greatest destruction of important nutrients. The enjoyable increase in flavour is really a measure of the breaking-down of complex substances within the food. By the same token, it is really not good to keep food hot for long after it has been cooked. The least possible delay between the pot and the plate is the ideal. A second cooking, even re-heating a soup on the second day, can greatly increase the destruction of health-sustaining properties. If you also freeze and thaw in between then the breakdown rate is further increased. It is a sad fact that soup that has been kept going for several days might taste wonderful, but its food value will be diminished every time it is re-heated.

Baking vegetables such as potatoes will break down their indigestible outer cellular structure, rendering them much more palatable. Starches, proteins and other complex nutrients are broken down during cooking, making them easier for your body to digest. This breakdown can increase the amount of nutrients that can be absorbed by your intestines that might otherwise pass through undigested. So although the micronutrients are partially destroyed by the heat, there will still be some useful nourishment there for your body. Not all minerals, trace elements and vitamins break down at the same rate and some are relatively stable during cooking, but overall most of these essential micronutrients will be compromised to a greater or lesser extent by heat. As a general rule the ideal diet contains raw salads, both raw and cooked vegetables and dried or fresh ripe sweet fruits.

For some food types careful pressure-cooking can work, and the emphasis here is on careful. It is too easy to overcook vegetables in a pressure cooker, but it can allow more of the goodness and the food's original flavour to be retained. This last is important where good digestion is the desired outcome, particularly as taste helps to prepare your digestive organs to deal with the kind of food being consumed. Greatly changing taste through a method of cooking or the addition of highly flavoured herbs or condiment flavouring can lead to indigestion for the reasons already mentioned. This may all seem a little tiresome, particularly if you enjoy your highly spiced dishes, but your digestive system will appreciate it.

Very high temperature cooking such as roasting, baking, frying, grilling and toasting can all cause considerable damage. If the food is a uniform mixture, such as bread, custard or a milk-pudding, the browning of the surface is not so serious; the interior is protected from the worst effects. If the food has a natural skin, this may be so scorched that most or all of the mineral and vitamin content, which is often concentrated close to the surface, is degraded.

Frying is particularly undesirable: partly because it leaves the food with at least a covering of fat, and often a considerable soaking into the bulk, which can easily disturb digestive efficiency; not least because the high temperature is bad for the fat itself and alters its substance. If frying is used, then any absorbent food should be first dipped in egg; this forms a seal almost instantly, keeping the fat out. If a frying pan is used—eg for omelettes—use no hotter than necessary to cook in a reasonable time. Higher temperatures alter the nature of the fat. If deep fat is used remember that each spell of cooking causes decomposition. What may have started off as relatively wholesome oil or fat soon becomes unwelcome to your digestive system.

Finally, casserole cookery, which many of the original food reformers regarded as the ideal method, their reasoning being that 'nothing is lost' because it all stays in the pot. Unhappily, as is so often the case, over-long cooking to 'bring out the flavour' often mars this apparent dietetic perfection. This over-cooking causes serious loss of nutrients through the decomposition and is further confused by the intermingling of the constituents of the food types.

Use of salt

Before the days of Teflon coatings many saucepans were made of aluminium, and there were serious health implications when cooking with salt. Now that most pans are coated with non-stick materials the use of aluminium utensils is mostly a thing of the past, the hazard of using salt in cooking is all about the amount you use. In general terms, anything above an absolute minimum for palatability is liable to cause disturbances in your body. Clinical observation has indicated a strong link between the quantity of salt you customarily take and the rapidity with which your tissues will age. More recent research in America has linked excessive salt intake and premature cell decay in all ages. Elasticity appears to be one of the principal casualties, and this is a vital property of healthy blood vessels. Anything that makes these less resilient leads to difficulty in maintaining adequate circulation. Hardening of the arteries in turn leads to problems in keeping the brain up to scratch; memory, concentration and the efficiency of hearing and eyesight may all show deterioration.

Long before these rather depressing conditions develop, an excess of salt can cause irritation to your digestive membranes, making you thirsty and sometimes resulting in raised blood pressure. It is too easy to maintain a craving for salt by drinking freely to slake the thirst produced by the previous intake of salt. Apart from interfering with good digestion, and over-burdening vital organs, excess fluid carries off essential mineral salts from the body in urine and perspiration. It creates an unwelcome vicious circle.

Whether ordinary commercial table salt, or sea salt, it should be used only in the strictest moderation. Uncooked foods should require none at all. Some cooked foods, such as eggs, are made more enjoyable by adding a little salt. The important word here is moderation.

Choice of utensils

Few of us use aluminium pots and pans these days but it is still important to avoid non-stick coated aluminium pans because scouring or scraping the surface of the pan destroys the protective coating.

Glass is ideal and modern cast iron with ceramic coatings are fine too. A material that occasionally causes trouble is enamelware, particularly if it is old or was originally made for any purpose other than cooking. Lead glaze was at one time widely used for enamels, and it can produce serious poisoning even in a brief contact with foodstuffs, especially if they are at all acidic. More modern enamel-ware should be perfectly safe. We are not talking here of the modern heavy cast iron pots that have an enamel coating, these are all completely safe as are earthenware intended for cooking, heat-resisting glass, fused silica and stainless steel. Although, of course, as you eat more and more of your foods raw you will use your pots and pans less and less.

Whilst the subject of toxic contamination has been raised, with modern pots, pans and crockery a far commoner cause of insidious poisoning these days is the careless use of detergents. These creep into the food on our plates via washing up liquids. You really must thoroughly rinse all cutlery, utensils, crockery and cookware in clean running water after washing-up. Failure to do so means that your crockery and cutlery have the potential to carry enough detergent to contaminate your next meal, and to cause serious and persistent digestive upsets. This is something that is often over-looked and certainly never mentioned in the adverts.

If you need to use detergent then use a bio-degradable one, and in moderation, and rinse well. If you use a dishwasher then you can use vinegar instead of rinse aid. Dishwashers should be kept clean.

Help your digestion

Your digestion generally works best when presented with uncomplicated foods, and least well when foods of contrasting category or type are combined. To understand why this should be, you will need to recognise the main food groups, and understand something of how and where your digestive system deals with them.

Food classification

We divide most foods quite simply into the following classes and percentages in which they should be consumed:

1 Carbohydrates (starches and sugars) and fats (vegetable and animal) 15 per cent by volume
2 Proteins (dairy foods, meat, nuts and pulses) 15 per cent by volume
3 The Cleansing Foods (salads, vegetables and fruit) 70 per cent by volume

4   Salts in moderation

5   Water in moderation

Carbohydrates, fats and oils

These are the 'energy' foods, of which sugars and starches (carbohydrates) and fats and oils (hydrocarbons) are the commonest. The carbohydrates range from the simplest sugars, which call for little or no digestive effort by the body, to complex vegetable fibre, or cellulose. This last is almost indigestible by any but the most vigorous human gut, relying heavily on an active bacterial population. And there are the intermediate starchy foods, which ought to start their digestion in your mouth, as a result of thorough chewing and mixing with your ptyalin-rich saliva. This works best in an alkaline or neutral medium, and can be inhibited by acids such as those found in some fruits and vegetables and all types of vinegar. In a good healthy gut your bacteria can break down the cellulose to release nutrients, when your gut is compromised these can be rendered unavailable.

So let's break down this group a little more.

1   Starches

For the most part these are found in traditional cereals, eg, wheat, oats, rye, rice, barley and maize as well as the more modern additions, quinoa, bulgar wheat and couscous. Tubers such as the potato and some root vegetables like carrot and parsnip have starch content. It is also the case that most of the cereals have a protein content that almost equals that of the starch.

As previously mentioned, the digestion of starch begins in your mouth by the action of your saliva, the more we chew our starches the more they become mixed up with saliva. This is why we recommend that they should be eaten as dry as possible. The saliva carries on its work until it becomes too acidified by the gastric juices in the stomach. Starch digestion stops when the condition becomes too acid, and the transformation of starch to sugar stops.

When the stomach contents pass into the duodenum they become alkaline again (or stay mildly acid) as the duodenum secretes a hormone that causes the gall bladder to release bile – a strongly alkaline substance – and the work of changing starch to sugar is resumed with the action of the pancreatic juices. These continue to break down any undigested starch and also break down the initial complex sugars into simpler ones. Enzymes from the intestinal wall complete the work and the carbohydrates have been transformed into glucose and fructose. These substances are either used or carried to the liver and stored as glycogen, where they stay until needed for energy. Normally the blood sugar rises slightly after a carbohydrate meal. The muscles take up substances that are carried by the blood; and the sugar is changed to glycogen and burned up to supply energy. Energy is used for both movement and heat production. When more energy is needed, the liver changes the stored glycogen into sugar and this is partly controlled by insulin, a secretion of the pancreas, and when this is deficient the concentration of sugar in the blood can rise to dangerous levels. This is when type 2 diabetes becomes evident, if you have a high sugar level then the duty falls on your kidneys to eliminate the excess sugar.

Carbohydrates not used immediately for energy can be changed in the body to fat and stored as adipose tissue. Carbohydrates are acid-forming foods.

2 Sugars

Apart from naturally occurring sugars in fruits and vegetables the main source of sugars in our food are cane sugar which is derived from cane and beet, and treacle, molasses and syrup which are all by-products of the manufacture of crystalline cane sugar. Honey is also a major source, and is much loved by health seekers. Lactose or milk sugar is an ingredient in many processed foods. More recently palm syrup has started to be widely used and its inclusion in many of the non-food snacks and fast foods has become questionable and controversial. The excess of fructose may be contributing to the massive rise in Type 2 diabetes. In Type 2 diabetes there is not enough insulin, or the insulin is inefficient, so the cells are only partially unlocked and sugars build up in the blood. So in the average diet, refined sugar in some form or another is the predominant sugar source, but to be made available to the body it has to be broken down. The difference is that the sugars found in fresh and dried fruit are ready for assimilation and are also associated with organised vitamins and minerals that the body recognises as nutritious. Highly refined sugar has no vitamin or mineral content, just calories.

3 Cellulose

This substance forms the cell walls of fruits and vegetables, and is present in the outer layers of cereals. It used to be thought that cellulose was quite impervious to human digestive juices. This is probably true of the harder, woody types, but the softer forms as found in the green leafy vegetables are more responsive to a healthy digestive system.

Undigested cellulose in the intestine is termed 'roughage' and its presence is considered beneficial to intestinal health. However, the practice of taking bran as your choice of roughage can be extremely harmful. Bran contains phytic acid, which joins up with calcium, as well as other essential minerals in your system. This forms an insoluble salt that leaves your body via the bowel. Bran therefore can run away with the calcium in your diet, and even from the tissues of your body, including your bones. This is another reason to eat starches in balance – even the goodies like wholemeal bread. If you are in the habit of eating soft, sloppy starches – such as porridge – your saliva is barely activated and the food does not get chewed so it arrives in the stomach with no pre-digestion, and this can allow them to be delivered to your intestines partially digested and ready to ferment giving you discomfort and flatulence.

4 Fats

Fats and oils are derived from both animal and vegetable sources. In the former group are butter, cheese, meat and bacon fat, milk, cooking fats such as lard, suet and dripping, in the latter, nut fat, seed oils and olive oil. Margarine is made both from nut fats and seed oils, although we do not generally recommend the use of margarine because it is a highly processed food. In butter the fat content is about 80 per cent, in cheese 30 per cent, in nuts 50–60 per cent. The function of fat is two-fold. It supplies energy, (twice as much as proteins and carbohydrates) and is needed for building vital substances (such as lecithin) that are essential for the composition of your cells and nervous tissue. We would recommend that you get your oils from vegetable, rather than animal sources. Most fats are not whole foods and have undergone some level of processing. These should be eaten is moderation and as unprocessed as possible. Extra virgin olive oil can help to retard the oxygenation of finely chopped or grated vegetables as well as assisting the uptake of vitamins in the gut.

The fats and oils pass through the stomach unchanged, the digestion of fats does not take place in the stomach but begins in the duodenum. Here only a small amount needs to be broken down, after this the remainder of the fat becomes emulsified and passes as fat through the intestinal wall. It is carried by the lymphatic system to the blood and from here it is passed into fat deposits, where it stays until required. Because of this delayed start to fat digestion, it is particularly undesirable to coat starchy foods with oils or fats, particularly as this can prevent the onset of starch digestion in the mouth.

Broadly there are three types of fat in the foods we eat; saturated fats, trans fats and unsaturated fat, they are all energy foods but trans fats should be avoided. They appear on food labels as hydrogenated fat, an ingredient in many cheap processed foods. Saturated fats are found in cheese, cream, meat products, baked goods and confectionery and should be eaten in moderation and can, if eaten in excess, have an adverse affect on your cholesterol levels. The last type is unsaturated fat and this is found in nuts, seeds, avocados, oily fish, olive oil, coconut butter and sunflower oil. In this group can be found the essential fatty acids. These are unsaturated fatty acids that are essential to human health, but cannot be manufactured in the body. They are of particular importance to the health of the nervous system. The unsaturated fats are the preferred type to include in your diet, with the proviso that all fats should be taken in balance with your overall food intake.

Because starches, sugars, oils and fats are acid-forming foods they should not form more than 30 per cent of the total of your food intake.

Proteins

Proteins are considered to be the 'building blocks' and supply the essential amino acids that are vital for our health, without protein nothing can live. But as adults we only need proteins to make up 15 per cent of our intake. Growing children will need a higher percentage. The main food sources of protein are:

1 Meat, poultry and fish.
2 Animal derived proteins such as cheese, eggs and milk.
3 Vegetables sources: legumes such as peas, beans, chickpeas and lentils; nuts of different types, and cereals. The latter often contain about 25 per cent proteins and 25 per cent carbohydrates in their makeup.

For the food-reformer, milk, cheese, eggs, nuts, peas, beans and lentils are the commonest sources of protein (with some real reservations about milk, that will be discussed later). All flesh foods, if you choose to include these in your diet, are rich in protein. But it is ironic that orthodox dieticians like to term meat proteins 'first class' and vegetable proteins 'second class'. This is an inversion of the simple biological fact that all animal protein that we find palatable to eat is derived from vegetables; therefore vegetable protein is primary, and animal secondary. Whichever of those protein rich foods you choose to balance your diet it is wise to buy organic and avoid unwanted prophylactic antibiotics and growth hormones.

Proteins are mainly digested in the stomach, in quite strongly acidic conditions. It will therefore make sense that to eat foods that prefer an alkaline condition for digestion, such as starches (bread, pastry, cereals) at the same time as those preferring acid, is likely to inhibit proper digestion and invite potential problems.

So many bouts of indigestion, and symptoms such as heartburn, result from these ubiquitous food combinations.

The function of proteins

How much protein should we eat and which kinds are best? Proteins are required mainly for growing in the younger years, and then building and repair throughout the rest of our life. Breast milk, which is a complete food for a rapidly growing baby, has only 2.7 per cent protein and the need for proteins throughout our lives tends to be much overrated. To make proteins available to the body they have to be broken down into simpler substances. This breaking down begins in the stomach, and continues in the first part of the small intestine, enzymes from the pancreas also play their part. The protein has now been transformed into amino acids, and these can be absorbed through the cell walls into the blood and lymph. From the circulating blood, each cell in the body takes up the acids it needs and rearranges them to build the kind of protein particular to itself. The original protein has been resolved into its constituent parts, transported around the body and then absorbed and reassembled into the combinations needed by different tissues.

The elimination of excess amino acids leads to the formation of urea that has to be excreted, mainly by your kidneys, but they also create extra work for the liver. If they are not expelled they can be deposited as uric acid crystals in your joints or other non-vital tissues. So a diet that is too high in protein can lead to trouble in your bowels and in your kidneys as well as unpleasant conditions such as gout. We suggest that the low-protein diet is desirable, and recommend that from 30–45 grams per day of mixed protein is the figure for reasonable health maintenance. This amount can be obtained from 120 grams of cooked lean meat or from 145 grams of cooked fish or 120 grams of cheese, 120 grams of dried pulses or four standard eggs. It is important to stress that the proteins must be obtained from a variety of sources. To eat four eggs a day would soon result in serious trouble. Indeed we recommend that no more than 2–3 eggs should be eaten weekly, this is mainly because the high sulphur content can be hard on already compromised kidneys. All proteins are acid-forming in your system.

The cleansing foods

'The cleansing foods' is a description that calls for some explanation. Whereas the first two food groups supply the immediate needs of the body for energy and tissue-maintenance, they give rise to acidic wastes and residues. The body must eliminate these speedily or all vital functions are impaired, if they are consumed in too great a quantity some essential functions can be severely disrupted. 'Elimination' here does not just mean opening of the bowels or urination, it is the complex process whereby the blood-purifying organs extract, or modify, and then excrete the acidic wastes that result from the assimilation and digestion of proteins. (Other foods are acid forming but protein is a major contributor.) The cleansing organs are your liver, kidneys, bowels, lungs and skin. The cleansing foods are characterised by their valuable contents of organised minerals, trace elements and vitamins, such as those that are found in unadulterated wholefoods, and these are essential for eliminative efficiency. Vitamins and minerals in their natural state, in real wholefoods, are living elements, and quite different to the laboratory cultured versions available in tablet or powder form. Your body will often tend to take up the synthetics first if the naturally occurring elements in your food are not immediately available. So, avoid the supplements, you will not need them if your diet is right.

This group of foods is much wider than the previous two, covering many differing varieties, but these may all be regarded as falling into two simple sub-divisions:

1   Fruits of most kinds.
2   Vegetables of all types.

And here we mention fresh milk again. At its very best raw organic milk could be regarded as a pre-digested form of fresh vegetables, with some of the benefits thereof. However, this is far from the case with the heat-treated and stale milk available on most supermarket shelves. The homogenised white liquid bears little resemblance to fresh live milk from a healthy mixed herd. If you cannot get organic raw milk then natural, unsweetened, organic yoghurt with live cultures is probably the best dairy alternative.

Fresh fruits and salad vegetables can all require considerable digestive effort from the body, but generally this is spread over a prolonged period, and there is no massive rush of blood to the stomach as occurs when a meal mostly made up of cooked protein is eaten. Cooked vegetables may also tend to draw blood away from the rest of the body and toward the digestive system. Even the many benefits of your midday salad, which allows your mind and body to be active even during digestion, can lose some of its healthful properties if too much cooked protein or carbohydrate is taken at the same time. These last two tend to rob your brain and muscles of blood during the early stages of active digestion. A balanced Nature Cure diet will automatically be low in both protein and carbohydrates, particularly if you follow the 70 per cent fruit and vegetables, 15 per cent proteins and 15 per cent carbohydrates ratios.

For those of us living in the Northern Hemisphere and in more temperate climates, some of the more acid fruits can present a bit of a problem. They are rarely properly ripened before picking and the acid content can be greater than fruits grown locally and picked sweet and fresh. Your taste buds should guide you, if the fruit is sweet and juicy it is probably fine in modest amounts, if it is tart or sour then it is probably best avoided. Apart from interfering with the digestion of starch, if taken at the same meal, tart, sour or unripe acid fruits usually remain un-neutralised for a considerable time.

Water and other liquids

Unnecessary drinking of water and other liquids is probably the commonest, well-intentioned error in most people's daily habits. Nature Cure practitioners work consistently against the popular belief that you should drink at least three pints of water a day, even if you have to force it down. Often this is on top of the other liquids you take in as coffee, tea, alcoholic and soft drinks etc. It might be difficult to convince you that moderation in liquids is the healthier option, and we have many good reasons for advocating what is sometimes, rather dauntingly, called dry feeding.

There is a simple explanation for the medical faith in copious drinking; many patients are on atrocious diets and, often on strong medication. If unwholesome foodstuff can be flushed out, and drugs kept diluted these unfortunate patient's chances of survival may be improved. And it is worth pointing out here that if you are on medication then a greater level of fluid intake might be needed to reduce the damaging effect of the drugs, that is, until we can wean you off the chemicals and on to a more balanced, healthier diet.

LIVE WELL. EAT WELL. BE WELL.

Why is excess fluid bad?

Excess fluid of any type begins its unhelpful processes in your mouth, particularly if you are in the habit of taking a mouthful of food followed immediately by a mouthful of liquid. This liquid dilutes the salivary enzymes and prevents the proper initial digestion of starches. In the stomach it again dilutes the juices, leading to delayed and inefficient digestion. This can cause the forms of fermentation and decomposition that can lead to heartburn and excessive flatulence. Other effects are perhaps slower to become obvious, but your heart, kidneys, muscular strength and physical toughness may also all suffer. On top of all that you are more likely to become overweight.

The links between salt and excessive thirst have already been touched upon, and with both salt and water the best amount is the least amount that will satisfy your taste and thirst. Real thirst is better slaked between meals, to lessen risk of the distresses listed above. Today, one is faced with an ever-diminishing choice of wholesome drinks. Genuine, fresh, unpasteurised buttermilk, beloved of early food reformers, is virtually extinct. Whole milk is almost universally heat-treated, making it untrustworthy for infants and unsuitable for adults. Should you be in the happy position of being able to purchase genuine, raw, organic fresh milk from a healthy mixed herd, then other protein-rich foods in your diet should be reduced accordingly.

One note of caution here with milk drinking in adults; milk is a complete food designed for a rapidly growing calf. It is full of proteins, micro-nutrients and natural growth hormones and just the foodstuff that cancerous growths will love.

Spring water may still be relatively pure, but well water and tap water have increasing amounts of contaminants such as chlorine, fluoride, nitrates, hormones and pesticides. Rainwater, collected off roofs, is even more undesirable because it tends to also include a wide range of airborne pollutants.

As far as possible, you should try to deal with your thirst by eating whole, fresh foods that are naturally juicy, and by avoiding spices and other thirst inducing processed or junk foods. Fruit juices are rarely as thirst quenching as the whole fruit and it is easy to take too much in one go. One glass can contain the juice of three or four whole fruits, which in their original form would take some time and effort to chew and digest. Juice drinks are full of sugar and artificial sweeteners, and the diluted juices are full of refined sugars.

Tea and coffee have many unwelcome constituents in addition to the burden of excess fluid, but the substitutes made from roasted grains, roots or fruits may be taken in modest quantity, and the occasional cup of decaffeinated coffee, provided that it has had the caffeine removed by the water technique, is also an acceptable drink. Decaffeination is usually achieved by the use of carbon tetrachloride, the same chemical that is used in dry-cleaning. Use a small cup rather than a mug because it is the first few sips that are the satisfying ones. Don't drink scalding hot liquids; wait until they have cooled a little.

Constituents

For some health conscious people it is very important to ensure that they know exactly what is in each item of food and what vitamins, minerals and trace elements are present. But this is to invest each item of food with too much individual importance. They eat two of this or three of that every day to ensure that they have the RDA (recommended daily allowance) of a particular vitamin or mineral. Ideally, the best thing is to have a balanced and varied diet that includes the main food types in reasonable proportions, and you don't need to eat every one every day. If you read Joanna Blythman's[1] excellent book *What to Eat* she covers all the information you might need. The interesting thing is that if you eat a wholefood diet, rich in vegetables, salad greens, fresh and dried fruits, nuts, pulses, fresh live yogurt and some unprocessed dairy and eggs then you will have all the building blocks your body will ever need. Calories are a useful tool to calculate your total daily intake, but they only record the energy released by burning up the particular foodstuff. They do not tell you the nutritional value. For information only, there is a chart of vitamins and minerals and the natural food sources for each at the end of this chapter. But it is not included so that you can obsess about every mouthful or each food item, but rather to illustrate that you can get everything you need from an honest balanced diet. Again, following the 70:15:15 per cent ratio of fresh fruits and vegetables: protein: carbohydrates will keep you right. If you are unwell then seek advice from your Nature Cure practitioner about your diet.

If you have chosen to follow a vegan or fruitarian diet then more care might be needed to ensure that you get enough of certain vitamins in your diet. In particular Vitamin B12 is virtually impossible to obtain from a completely plant based diet, this is only needed in very small amounts and because of this it can take some time to show up as lacking, but when it does it will affect you nervous system. Getting your quota of B12 is vital to your wellbeing. Natural sources are eggs, dairy products, liver, kidney and other meats. It is also present in yeast flakes, yeast extract and some fermented foods, but these should be consumed in moderation. There is conflicting research about the use of spirulina as a source. Otherwise, none of the animal products are naturally included in vegan or fruitarian diets, therefore some type of supplement might need to be taken, particularly if the idea of using a natural animal derived source is unacceptable to you.

Of course, some of you will have other dietary needs or preferences, and proportions of certain food types might need to be increased or reduced or these foods may need to be cut out completely. The important thing with your food is to get it 'about right' and stop worrying. If you are healthy and active you can enjoy your varied fruit breakfast, your lovely crunchy raw salad lunch and simple evening meals. If you cannot take your salad to work and have to eat from the canteen, then have your cooked meal in the middle of the day and your salad in the early evening.

But how do you get it 'about right'? The following information is intended as a set of guidelines and is not set in stone; you can experiment to find the best computations for your lifestyle. Your Nature Cure practitioner will be able to advise you about your best way forward.

Some simple guidelines:

1 Base your diet on 70 per cent salads, vegetables (raw and conservatively cooked) and fruit.
2 Eat wholefoods – avoid processed foods.
3 Eat organic.
4 Eat calmly, in a pleasant environment and enjoy your mealtimes.
5 Don't be obsessive – worry is a waste of valuable energy.

Mealtime suggestions

Breakfasts

Apart from omitting it altogether, the Nature Cure food reformer has three main choices of breakfast:

1 Fruit only; fresh, dried (soaked or unsoaked) or a mixture of the two.
2 A small salad, with or without bread or biscuit.
3 Starchy, with prepared cereal or bread as basis.

The first two are obviously more likely to be favoured in the warmer months, the third in wintertime. As a drink, a small glass of koumiss or fresh organic milk – about a quarter of a pint (140ml) – is compatible with any of the options, as is a couple of tablespoonfuls of active live yogurt. On cold mornings a small cup – not a great big mug full – of coffee-substitute or water washed decaffeinated coffee is acceptable with a starchy meal. Eat the starchy foods first and chew well and have your hot drink at the end of the meal and drink it slowly.

For growing children, a more substantial breakfast is needed, and cereal with dried fruit, followed by bread or toast, would be ideal. Once or twice per week, for a change, an egg, scrambled, poached or boiled can be added.

More generally, it is better to avoid too many kinds of fruit at one time. One variety of dried fruit and one of fresh is sensible. For instance four medium-sized stewed prunes and a fresh apple should be an adequate quantity. You can of course have many different combinations. For example, two or three dried figs and a pear, a tablespoon of raisins (soaked overnight) with a fresh peach or apricot. It will be dependent on what fresh fruit is available as the year progresses.

Bread should be genuine wholemeal or partially made from spelt wheat. It should be organic and stone ground out of preference. If you cannot find this product locally consider purchasing a bread maker, or get creative and make your own loaf. If you choose to eat your bread toasted it should be allowed to cool before buttering. Cereal should be wholegrain, preferably not from maize or polished rice and without added sugar and should be eaten as dry as possible and chewed well. Over time you will find that a small portion, taken dry and thoroughly chewed, will develop a better flavour and give more satisfaction than a greater quantity gulped down with milk and sugar. Muesli is a good alternative to processed packet cereals and can be eaten with dried fruit and yogurt in moderate amounts.

Dried fruits go with bread or cereal – these are both carbohydrates – but most fresh fruits do not, due to the acid content of the fruit. The exception here is banana; depending on how ripe the fruit is the starch content can be as much as 25 per cent, the balance being mainly sugars.

Salad should be enough in itself, but if you are in a more active occupation then there may be a need for something extra, a slice of wholemeal bread or toast, or a crispbread biscuit, is suitable. If time is limited, fruit is preferable to salad, since the latter requires really thorough chewing for proper utilisation whereas fruit is a little easier on the digestion.

Lunchtime salads

For you to achieve a balanced and adequate diet, a considerable proportion of fresh fruits and uncooked vegetables need to be included. Although it might not be practicable for you to eat a totally unfired, or raw, diet it can have many points in its favour.

One of the knock-on advantages of all the chewing you do with raw food is sound, strong teeth as well as the improvement in your general health. Cooked food is too easy to swallow with little chewing and this means that often it doesn't get properly digested and the utilisation of the nutrients is compromised. Nuts, too, can be eaten in excessive quantities when milled down and softened by cooking, whereas if they are eaten uncooked, they require you to do the work of the milling machine.

For those of you who have been used to a mainly cooked and otherwise processed diet is it important to make a regular feature of salads. Their value can hardly be over-stressed, especially where acid-forming starches and proteins have predominated. Salads have the supreme advantage of presenting their organised minerals and vitamins undiminished and undamaged by cooking.

However, these benefits are not enjoyed without effort; particularly if you are not used to eating a lot of raw foods, and initially it might be quite daunting. There is a saying: 'Take nothing into the mouth but solids; swallow nothing but liquids,' this is excellent advice. Take your time over your meal, include a nice rainbow of different coloured vegetable and salads, this will make it so much more enjoyable especially on a grey winter's day. Breathing through your nose while chewing can also help to prepare your digestion; the natural flavours and aromas of foods are powerful peptic stimulants.

Most salads should ideally be eaten without highly spiced or flavoured dressings, but a little olive or other seed oil can help with the digestion of green leafy vegetables. Make a simple dressing using olive oil and a little lemon juice, or tamari, and use it sparingly.

Malt or spirit vinegars should be avoided and mayonnaise should be homemade.

It can be argued that where salads contain shredded or grated vegetables, an acid or oily dressing will protect against rapid oxidation and vitamin loss. The ideal, however, is to avoid both delay and too much dressing.

Soups

Fresh vegetable soups, properly prepared, form a palatable and nourishing addition to a meal. They are rich in organised salts (minerals in a form which can be readily assimilated by the body) and a variety of vitamins. However, overcooking can greatly reduce their food value, because organised salts and vitamins are susceptible to oxidation and decomposition with prolonged heating.

Ordinarily, soup should not be eaten every day; alternate days are often enough. If you are the type of cook who likes to put time and effort into preparing a delicious soup, it may be discouraging to be told that second-day soup, which so often is even tastier than the fresh version, is not dietetically desirable. In the winter months a baked jacket potato every other day can be an ideal accompaniment to your salad.

Soup should only take 10–15 minutes to make if you grate the vegetables and potatoes then liquidise them. For a more hearty soup with larger pieces of vegetable and potato, cooking time should take no more than 15–20 minutes. It is usually digested better if taken slowly, and with something chewy such as toasted wholemeal bread or a crusty wholemeal roll.

Good soup does not require meat or bone stock. If starting from scratch, a modest addition of rice or barley adds body to a soup but these ingredients will considerably increase the cooking time. If vegetable water has been kept from a previous meal, this gives a far more wholesome and nutritious stock than water from boiled bones or meat scraps. (However, 24 hours is about the limit of useful life of vegetable water.) Some use yeast-extract, or concentrated vegetable extract as basic seasoning, but these can be easily over-used, swamping the natural flavours of the fresh ingredients.

If butter or margarine is used in soup, add just before serving. Salt should be avoided or if essential then use the least amount that will give you an acceptable flavour. Any seasoning should be added toward the end of cooking, and when fresh vegetable stock is used the addition of salt should be unnecessary. As your taste buds adjust to more raw and unprocessed foods your need for seasoning will lessen.

Vegetables and vegetable dishes

Unless you are in exceptionally good health and can eat raw for every meal, most people have a real need for some cooked foods, as well as salads. Vegetables in particular can pose a serious problem for the less-than-vigorous digestion unless their fibrous texture has been partially broken down by cooking.

If fruits are not taken for breakfast they can be used as desserts. In this scheme, dairy produce appears (a) as cheese with salad, (b) as eggs or cheese in savouries or sauces, and (c) as milk for drinking in small amount or as an ingredient in cooked dishes.

If you change to a completely unfired diet in adult life you run the risk of inadequate nutrition. This may show less in your body bulk than in your emotional and nervous state. If you are lacking a really robustly active gut that can cope easily with the digestion of vegetable tissues, then your mental stability and confidence may be diminished. For the majority, some cooked food and some dependence on organic dairy produce is desirable. These are certainly to be taken in preference over the processed created proteins made from soya or fungi. Basically, cooking should always be to the least amount that makes the food acceptable and enjoyable. Vegetables should be exposed to high temperature for the shortest practicable time, using the least amount of water, and not chopped or sliced smaller than necessary (except for soup). The water in which the vegetables have been cooked is not the elixir some would have us believe, but it can be a good basis for other dishes such as sauces and soups, provided that it is kept for no more than 24 hours and always in the fridge.

As explained in connection with utensils, salt should be used only sparingly in cooking, and the use of pepper should also be limited, as it has the potential to be damaging to your liver. Culinary herbs, fresh or dried, can add interest and variety, but can easily be over-used. The flavour of the dish becomes that of the herb, and this can be bad news for digestive efficiency. The aim of the food reformer is to move toward a fuller appreciation of natural flavours. At first these may be faint and elusive, sometimes even downright unappetising if you are used to highly flavoured junk foods, but familiarity and an improving sense of taste and texture should bring growing enjoyment. It is well worth sticking with it.

The pulses: dried peas, beans and lentils, are often over-used in vegetarian cookery. These foods, like nuts, are concentrated, yet relatively low in vitamins, but they are still a better source of protein than fish or meat weight for weight. Fresh peas and beans, by contrast are living vegetables. Naturally dried peas and beans and some seeds can be brought back to the living state by being soaked and allowed to germinate. After basic germination they

LIVE WELL. EAT WELL. BE WELL.

are right for cooking. Some are even better grown in a sprouter for a few days; the sprouts can then be used as salad vegetables. Pressure-cooking the pulses from dry loses this valuable opportunity.

Dried pulses and nuts made up into highly spiced cooked dishes are really the blight of popular vegetarianism. Feeling yourself denied your usual animal proteins it is easy to over eat vegetable based proteins when they are in the form of processed burgers and veggie mince. With a little less reliance on proteins, and a growing understanding of the properties of fresh vegetables, the result will be a much better balance. When pulses are used, one simple way of helping to redress their acidic tendency is to use onions with them. For savouries, the two go well together, both dietetically and in flavour.

Savouries

Savouries, although delicious, should not really form the main part of the meal. They should be interesting additions to the real stars, the vegetables, which will take up 70 per cent of your plate. Many made-up savouries can be faulted, according to food-reform principles, because of their combination, or mingling, of different kinds of foods. For example mixing proteins and starches, such as cheese and breadcrumbs. Although for the true food combining enthusiast the mixture is technically indefensible, such 'lapses' become much less important if you keep savouries as a whole in their proper perspective. After all, they are not intended to be your main nourishment.

However, if you do want to make a meal out of the savoury, it is best to avoid incompatible mixtures of ingredients. A dish composed mainly of beans or eggs, with cheese, is better than one of flour and cheese coated with cooking fat; the first is almost all protein, while the second has three distinctly different constituents. Vigorously healthy people appear to be unaffected by regularly eating such combinations, but there is no guarantee that will always be the case. Interestingly, sometimes it is the person who has a sensitive or 'complaining' stomach who is in the better long-term situation as they are warned early of any digestive difficulties and can adjust their diet accordingly.

If you have persistent stomach or gut upsets you would be well advised to avoid fried foods, and if you suffer with a chronic acid conditions such as rheumatism you should be careful to avoid high-protein intake as well.

Desserts

Fresh or dried fruit, cooked or uncooked, is probably the ideal dessert. In most cases it is advisable to avoid fresh, acid fruits at the same meal as bread, biscuits or other starchy food. For the majority, even those with a robust digestive system, acid and starch can be a distressing combination. So no more rhubarb crumble and custard! Tasty it might be, but sadly dietetically speaking it's a nightmare.

The principal acid fruits are: oranges, lemons, grapefruit, cooking apples and most varieties of stone fruits and berries. The fruits most in harmony with starchy foods are the dried versions of prunes, figs, dates, raisins, apricots, peaches, pears and apples. Also tolerable for most people at the end of a meal containing starches are fresh peaches, sweet apples, pears, apricots and grapes. Melon should ideally be eaten on its own.

Bananas, as we get them in temperate countries, are picked while still unripe, and they ripen partially in the hull of a boat.

This means that they are lacking their natural complement of sunshine and this renders them largely starchy and low in minerals and vitamins. What are regarded as 'over-ripe' bananas may have a considerable proportion of their starch converted to sugar, but this hardly improves their dietetic value. Bananas are beloved of athletes because their potassium content can help to prevent cramp; that may be but they can easily induce heartburn in those with sensitive stomachs. Sun-dried bananas are in a different class and in this form are as acceptable as the other dried fruits listed above.

Canned and bottled fruits do not compare with fresh, except in taste and colour and if bottled fruit is not protected from light they can lose more food value. Frozen fruits may provide some welcome variety in the winter months, but they too will have lost a considerable amount of their original goodness.

Miscellaneous suggestions

Avoid eating when tired. Digestion of food is one of the hardest tasks faced by the body, and it is not fair to make heavy demands when it is exhausted. Better to miss a meal and rest, but if that seems too drastic, make it a very light meal, maybe of a single food type, if possible uncooked or only gently steamed or boiled.

At mealtimes it is best to eat the salads and vegetables first, before the starches and proteins. This does two things; it means you are less likely to overeat and if you take your time you will also get a better feedback from your stomach when it is full.

It should be recognised that a relatively small excess of one particular food type can upset the balance of an otherwise well-selected diet. As a general rule, the foods that are digested most rapidly are those ones that produce the greatest acid residue; the alkalising foods digest comparatively slowly. Therefore if the appetite is satisfied with an excess of starches, sugars, fats or proteins, the digestive activity will tend to diminish before the salads and vegetables in your meal are properly dealt with. This is the situation in which these vital living foods can become little more than 'roughage', a fibrous mass, filling your bowels.

Remember that your digestive organs need to rest sometimes. They should be able to benefit from sleep just as other bodily members. This is why we suggest that the evening meal should be eaten early, and that nothing much if anything should be taken before bedtime. If there is a real feeling of need for something at that time, a piece of fresh fruit is probably the easiest on your system.

Mealtimes should be happy times. They are not the place for resolving family or work relationship problems.

A few dos and don'ts

1   Follow the 70 per cent salad, fruit and vegetables, 15 per cent proteins and 15 per cent carbohydrates guideline. You can't go far wrong if you do.
2   Eat organically produced or home grown food whenever possible.
3   Don't make drastic changes to your diet without guidance from a Nature Cure practitioner.
4   Eat no more than three simple meals per day, with nothing in between.
5   If any digestive discomfort follows a meal, omit the next one.
6   Keep your meals simple: fruit breakfast, salad lunch and cooked vegetable evening meal, for example.
7   Avoid eating late in the evening.

8   Eat only a simple single food type meal if you are really tired after a busy day, or skip it altogether if you are upset about something.

9   Don't become obsessed about your food, try the mantra: 'Get your food as right as you can, and then enjoy it.'

What is koumiss?

To avoid any confusion, here are a few notes on what we call 'Koumiss'. The Kingston Clinic's version was made from unpasteurised organic milk from a local mixed herd of cows. The milk – minus the thickest of the cream – was put into a shallow covered vessel in a warm place, it was regularly aerated by whisking. After a few days the milk would 'sour' as microorganisms proliferated and the result was a thin version of yoghurt with a sharp fresh taste. If it tasted at all rancid, it would be discarded and a new batch started afresh. It is currently impossible to legally obtain raw milk in Scotland and therefore true Koumiss is hard to make north of the border. There are suppliers of raw milk in England and it should be possible to make good Koumiss without a starter culture provided that the milk is genuinely raw and fresh.

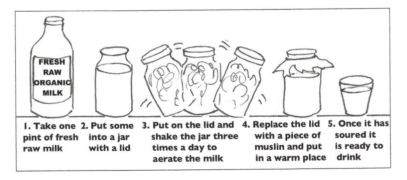

FRESH RAW ORGANIC MILK				
1. Take one pint of fresh raw milk	2. Put some into a jar with a lid	3. Put on the lid and shake the jar three times a day to aerate the milk	4. Replace the lid with a piece of muslin and put in a warm place	5. Once it has soured it is ready to drink

An alternative method to make a small amount of koumiss is to put the milk into a wide necked jar and secure the lid for shaking and agitation. Once this is done the lid should be removed and replaced with muslin. Of course, the lid should be put back on each time the souring milk is being shaken and aerated and the muslin replaced after the exercise. The jar should be kept in a warm place.

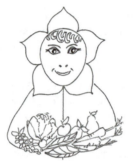

References

1 Washington State University. Published in the British Journal of Nutrition. 15.07.2014.
2 Blythman, Joanna 'What to Eat' 2009.

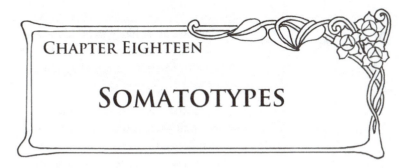

CHAPTER EIGHTEEN

SOMATOTYPES

IT WAS AMERICAN psychologist William Herbert Sheldon who devised the Somatotype classifications for human body shape. It was his attempt to explain simply the reasons for the different bone size and muscle bulk in individuals, and also why some people put on weight easily while others struggle to gain it. His study involved 4,000 university students in the 1940s. The system in a variety of forms is still in use today.

He divided the human physique into three basic types each one relating to the three different layers of embryonic development. The endoderm develops into the digestive tract, the mesoderm into the muscle, heart and blood vessels and the ectoderm into the skin and nervous system. The three categories are:

ENDOMORPHS: At this end of the scale the individual is built around their gut, they have a large frame, carry a high percentage of body fat, with wide hips but narrower shoulders. In the females the ankles and wrists tend to be slim. They are not always fat, but often curvaceous. They find it hard to lose weight, and hard to maintain the weight loss if they do. Entertaining, food and company are essential to their happiness.

MESOMORPHS: Those in the middle of the scale have muscular bodies with wide shoulders, narrow hips and strong limbs.

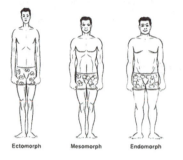

Ectomorph   Mesomorph   Endomorph

They are more likely to build muscle, than store fat, but they also find it easy to lose the extra. They tend to be athletic, sporty people.

ECTOMORPHS: Those at the ectomorphic end of the scale tend to be slender and lean, they have narrow frames with long arms and legs, their faces are thin and they have high foreheads. They carry little of no fat and rarely put on weight; they also have little extra muscle. Fashion models are usually ectomorphs, but so are many academic types, the ones who tend to live in their heads.

There has been a tendency over the years to make the body types into cultural stereotypes. For instance, the endomorphs are thought of as slow, untidy, and lazy and love food, company and communication. Mesomorphs were considered to be well liked and industrious, adventurous with a love of taking risks, brave and sometimes dominant. Ectomorphs are seen as intelligent, but nervous types often drawn to solitary sports such as marathon running with a tendency to be introverted.

It is rare for a person to be only one type and most of us have characteristics of all three groups. Sheldon described each group as being on a scale of 1–7 with the most extreme in each type scoring 7 and the least extreme being a 1. So a person who scores 4–4–4 has a better chance of being reasonably well balanced both physically and mentally as well as in their activity levels, than someone for instance scoring 7–1–1 or 1–7–1. But this system can only ever be a rule of thumb and is only one useful tool to assess

LIVE WELL. EAT WELL. BE WELL.

body types as part of an overall approach that must take in all the aspects of an individual's make-up.

Eating for your body type

So what does this have to do with eating for your body type? Looking at the three types goes some way towards explaining why some people can apparently eat whatever they want, and stay slim, while others, despite their best efforts, struggle to keep the fat off. There is some evidence that the gut lengths within the three types are different too. The Endomorphs, having the longest gut length, risk food being delayed in transit and so starting to putrefy. For them, avoiding meat and fish and eating a plant based diet is important, they thrive on low calorie food and are well served by a predominantly raw diet. Deprived of food they are miserable, and without company they tend to eat to compensate, and so are likely to put on more extra weight. At the other end of the scale the Ectomorph is less likely to be so interested in food, they have a shorter gut length and are prone to, as one practitioner put it, 'intestinal hurry'. They are happy in isolation, their inherent nervous energy means that they don't lay down fat. They can sometimes struggle on a completely raw diet, although psychologically they would be drawn to it, and some cooked food is sensible for these individuals to help to keep them grounded. The Mesomorphs are in the middle, they can eat pretty much what they want if they exercise it off, and if they do gain weight, they find it relatively easy to shed it again. They can perform well on a plant based diet with some dairy for protein and vitamins.

Your practitioner will work with you to devise the diet that best suits your 'type', but as usual sticking to the 70:15:15 balance is a good guide. The difference will be in the preparation of the food and overall amounts. It might seem like a good thing if you never put on weight and can apparently eat all sorts of junk food without gaining weight. But the body still has to deal with the wastes and has to store them somewhere and this is often in the joints. Over time, some chronic impairment of movement can result. If you lay down fat easily, at least you get a quick warning – if you choose to heed it – that your diet is out of balance, and you can cut out the problem foods and give your body a good chance of keeping healthy. In the middle group you may find that in youth you can eat whatever you want and stay slim but as the years pass this can change and in middle age you start to put on weight. This may mean that you need to make a few adjustments in the balance, volume and type of the foods in your diet.

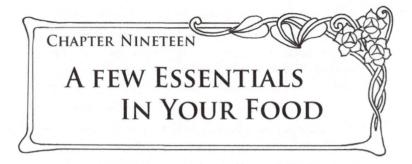

CHAPTER NINETEEN

A FEW ESSENTIALS IN YOUR FOOD

IN AN IDEAL, organic, balanced diet the range of essential vitamins and minerals should not be difficult to find. We need these elements to supply our bodies with the essential nutrition to allow healthy function. Following the advice to 'Eat a Rainbow' can go some way to ensuring that we get what we need. What follows is a general guide to what we need, what we need them for and which foods they are in.

CALCIUM (Ca) is the most abundant mineral in the body. It is in bones and teeth and is essential to every muscle movement and to our acid base equilibrium. For proper absorption from food it needs hydrochloric (stomach) acid, vitamins D (which you get from sunshine, so take every opportunity in the winter to get as much sun as you can in our Northern climes), A and C, phosphorus, magnesium and protein. Phytic acid and oxalic acid (found in spinach) can inhibit calcium absorption. Sugar also disturbs the calcium/phosphorus balance. Calcium is in milk and other dairy products, sesame seeds, soya beans, peanuts, green leafy vegetables, walnuts, almonds, brazil nuts, tofu, dried figs, corn tortillas and sunflower seeds.

PHOSPHORUS (P) is the second most abundant mineral in the body. Phosphorus is essential for biological action at a cellular level. It helps to convert glucose to glycogen and to synthesise phospholipids that transport fats around the body. Fats are essential to nerve impulse function. It works with calcium to maintain the phosphorus/calcium balance in your cells. It is in eggs, whole grains, nuts and seeds. It is also in meat and fish.

POTASSIUM (K) some five per cent of the total mineral content in the body is potassium and it works with sodium to create the sodium/potassium 'pump' maintaining the alkaline/acid balance in the body. It promotes the disposal of body/tissue waste and helps to supply oxygen to the brain. It is in brown rice, nuts, parsnip, potatoes, green leafy vegetables and bananas.

SODIUM (Na) is found in extracellular fluid and it works with potassium to maintain the osmotic pressure at the cellular level. Sodium also helps to keep other minerals soluble. Sodium chloride (table salt) is not ideal and needs to be used very sparingly. Better sources are: kelp, beets, carrots and chard.

MAGNESIUM (Mg) is present in the body in our bones with calcium and phosphorus and it helps to regulate our heartbeat. It assists with muscle contractions and helps to protect the nerves. It binds to milk and if we drink milk fortified with vitamin d it can be excreted from the body leading to deficiency. Refined white flour and sugar cause the body to use up stored magnesium to metabolise them and this too can lead to deficiency. Magnesium is found in: kelp, almonds, cashew nuts, brazil nuts, brown rice, soya beans and green leafy vegetables.

Trace element deficiencies

TRACE ELEMENT DEFICIENCIES are common partly as a result of conventional intensive agricultural practices, food processing and food choices. They can be corrected by eating the right foods. Recommended daily amounts differ widely from one person to another – for example, some illness may require increased amounts of a particular trace element to balance out the deficiency.

IRON (Fe) is the most abundant metallic trace element in the body; it is, amongst other things, essential for red blood cells which transport oxygen around the body. The richest source is in liver, but it is also found in: oatmeal, raisins, prunes, egg yolks, dried beans and green leafy vegetables.

ZINC (Zn) can often be low in vegetarians or people on low protein diets. Zinc takes a part in carbohydrate metabolism and is vital to fertility. Dietary sources are: pumpkin seeds, mushrooms, dried legumes, pecan nuts, brazil nuts, egg yolk and oats.

COPPER (Cu) is an abundant trace element and helps in the absorption of iron. But it is only needed in very small amounts and accumulations, or small excesses, can be damaging which is only one good reason for not drinking water out of the hot tank! Copper is in: soya beans, legumes, whole wheat, prunes and molasses.

There are many other trace elements and micronutrients that we need and can find in a healthy balanced organic diet. Of equal importance is regular daily exercise and deep breathing to ensure a sufficient supply of oxygen to allow the body to metabolise these essential micronutrients. There is one vitamin that needs a special mention:

VITAMIN B12 Although all vitamins are essential to good health and the proper functioning of the body, vitamin B12 deserves a particular mention. It can be lacking in extreme vegetarian, vegan or fruitarian diets and its lack, or inability of the body to utilise it, can cause nervous problems and anaemia. B12 is also essential for the synthesis of DNA and has a special importance for red blood cells. Food sources include liver and kidney, meat, eggs and dairy products. Vegans may need to have injections of B12 to ensure they have enough of this essential vitamin.

So if you have a diet rich in whole grains, green leafy vegetables, root vegetables, a little garlic and onion, avocado, fresh and dried stone fruits, sprouted seeds, legumes, brassicas, some organic eggs, butter and cheese, a little peanut butter, nuts, citrus fruits, fresh local fruits, some brown rice and a few potatoes – as well as a little of what you fancy – you are going to get all the nutrients you need from your food. If you are reasonably healthy your body will be able to extract all the vitamins, minerals and trace elements it needs.

VITAMINS	NATURAL FOOD SOURCES
Vitamin A Retinol	Carrots, Beetroot, Peaches, Apricots, Yams, Sweet Potato, Egg, Milk & Dairy.
Vitamin B1 Thiamine	Green and Yellow Vegetables, Peas, Beans, Lentils, Brown Rice, Bran, Whole Grains, Peanuts, Fruit & Milk.
Vitamin B2 Riboflavin	Green Leafy Vegetables, Cereals, Milk, Dairy, Egg, Fish.
Vitamin B3 Niacin	Avocado, Dates, Figs, Prunes, Egg, Peanut Butter, RawWheat Germ, Brewer Yeast, Liver & Fish.

LIVE WELL. EAT WELL. BE WELL.

VITAMINS	NATURAL FOOD SOURCES
Vitamin B5 Pantothenic Acid	Beans, Whole Grains, Nuts, Molasses, Royal Jelly, Meat, Brewer's Yeast.
Vitamin B6 Pyridoxine	Raw Wheat Germ, Cabbage, Milk, Egg, Liver, Kidney, Brewer's Yeast.
Vitamin B12 Cyanocobalamin	Egg, Dairy Products, Spirulina, Liver, Kidney & Meat.
Vitamin B15 Pangamic Acid	Brown Rice, Whole Grains, Pumpkin Seeds, Sesame Seeds.
Vitamin B17 Laetrile or Amygdalin	Stone Fruits, such as Apricot or Prunes.
Vitamin B9 Folic Acid	Green Leafy Vegetables, Carrots, Avocado, Beans, Egg Yolk, Pumpkin, Cantaloupe Melon & Liver.
Vitamin B7 Biotin	Brown Rice, Nuts, Egg Yolk, Fruits & Milk.
Vitamin B4 Choline	Green Leafy Vegetables, Egg Yolk, Brewer's Yeast, Broccoli, Shitake Mushrooms, Scallops.
Vitamin B8 Inositol	Peanut Butter, Cantaloupe Melon, Molasses, Wheat Germ, Organ Meats, Brewer's Yeast.
Vitamin C Ascorbic Acid	Whole Citrus Fruits, Broccoli, Peppers, Tomatoes, Green Leafy Vegetables, Melons, Yams, Potatoes.

VITAMINS	NATURAL FOOD SOURCES
Vitamin D	Sunshine, Dairy, Butter, Cheese, Oily Fish.
Vitamin E	Leafy Green Vegetables, Lettuce, Nuts, Seeds, Wholegrains, Egg, Raw Wheat Germ, Vegetable Oils.
Vitamin K1, 2 & 3 are made in the gut	Alfalfa, Green Leafy Vegetables, Broccoli, Yogurt, Buttermilk, Safflower & Soya Oil, Fish Liver.
Vitamin P	Citrus Fruits, Grapes, Plums, Blackcurrants, Apricots, Cherries, Blackberries.
MINERALS	NATURAL FOOD SOURCES
Calcium (Ca)	Green Leafy Vegetables, Sesame Seeds, Walnuts, Sunflower Seeds, Peanuts & Milk.
Phosphorus (P)	Whole Grains, Nuts, Seeds, Egg & Meat.
Potassium (K)	Green Leafy Vegetables, Citrus Fruits, Potatoes, Bananas, Tomatoes & Pineapple.
Sodium (Na)	Table Salt, Beets, Carrots, Chard, Dandelion Greens, Shellfish.
Magnesium (Mg)	Figs, Nuts, Apples, Green Leafy Vegetables, Raw Wheat Germ.
Sulphur (S)	Eggs.
Chlorine (Cl)	Kelp, Alfalfa & Fish.

TRACE ELEMENTS	NATURAL FOOD SOURCES
Iron (Fe)	Oatmeal, Dried Peach & Apricot, Raisins, Prunes, Eggs, Dried Beans, Green Leafy Vegetables, Liver & Kidney.
Zinc (Zn)	Mushrooms, Pumpkin Seeds, Egg Yolk, Dried Legumes, Milk, Mustard Seeds, Brazil Nuts & Raw Oysters.
Copper (Cu)	Legumes, Whole Wheat, Prunes, Soya Beans, Molasses, Liver & Seafood.
Manganese (Mn)	Nuts, Whole Grains, Green Leafy Vegetables, Peas, Clover, Ginger & Tea.
Chromium (Cr)	Raw Wheat Germ, Brewer's Yeast, Molasses, Meat & Shellfish.
Iodine (I)	Onions, Kelp, Seaweed & Shellfish.
Selenium (Se)	Raw Wheat Germ, Onions, Nuts, Seeds & Tuna.
Fluorine (Fl)	Kelp & Sea Foods.
Silica (Si)	Oats, Millet, Barley, Onions, Whole Wheat & Red Beets.
Molybdendum (Mo)	Legumes, Whole Grain Cereals, Dark Green Leafy Vegetables.
Germanium (Ge)	Garlic & Comfrey.
Boron (B)	Fruits & Vegetables.

TOXIC ELEMENTS	TO BE AVOIDED!
Lead	Environmental, Eating Calcium and Iron containing foods can help to prevent absorption of lead.
Mercury	Shark, Swordfish, King Mackerel & High Fructose Corn Syrup.
Cadmium	Shellfish, Liver & Kidney.

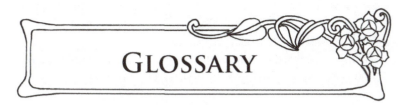

GLOSSARY

ACID WASTES

Products of metabolism that are carried by the blood. Proteins, tea and coffee create more acid wastes than salads, vegetables and fruit.

ACIDOSIS

Occurs when the blood has to continue carrying too much acid wastes after the cleansing organs cannot deal with the overload.

CAUSE AND EFFECT

The philosophical concept of causality. It is the relationship between events or things, where one is the result of the other. It is a combination of action and reaction.

CLEANSING ORGANS

The kidneys, liver, lungs, skin and bowels. They all have their part to play in dealing with the waste products of metabolism.

COLD COMPRESS

The application of a cold wet cotton cloth with a woollen covering. Most often used around the waist.

COLD SPLASH

The application of cold water using cupped hands, usually to the pelvic floor and low back.

CONGESTION

Usually a localised condition where there is an accumulation of blood or wastes obstructing the tissues; the state of being blocked with mucus.

CONSTITUTION

The inherited and acquired properties of your body. Lindlahr divided these into three planes of being — physical, mental and spiritual.

GLOMERULI

A network of capillaries located in the kidney. They perform the first stage in the filtering of waste products from the blood before these are carried out by the nephron and excreted in urine.

HEALING CRISIS

A healing crisis is an acute effort to rid the body of an overload of toxic wastes in the tissues. It results from the inherent healing forces dealing with the disease conditions. It is a positive and constructive activity.

HEALING FORCES

The positive forces in the body that tend towards recovery and good health.

HOMEOSTASIS

The balancing and control of internal conditions, including temperature and specific blood conditions in the body.

IATROGENESIS OR IATROGENIC also known as LATROGENESIS OR LATROGENIC

Inadvertent and preventable induction of disease or complications by the medical treatment or procedures of a physician or surgeon.

INTELLIGENT LEAVING ALONE

The acceptance that the body is in control and 'knows' what it is doing during a Healing Crisis and allowing the processes to proceed unhindered.

INTERFERENCE

Taking medication, or food when it is not needed for instance during a healing crisis.

LAW OF RETURN

The rule that organic gardeners and farmers obey, which demands that whatever is taken out of the soil is put back 'in equal measure'. If you take out vegetables, you would put in humus rich compost and manure in return.

LIFE-FORCE

Life is a primary force, an active principle forming part of any living thing. It is a part of our physical vitality.

MUSCLE TONE

The continuous and passive partial contraction of a muscle, that helps to maintain posture.

PRE-EXISTING CONDITION

This is the state of your tissues before symptoms appear (rather than the American medical insurance definition) that can offer a suitable host to viruses or bacteria. See Toxaemia below.

PSYCHOSOMATIC

Of both the mind (psycho) and the body (soma) working in tandem. So for instance, a physical illness, or other condition caused or aggravated by a mental factor such as emotional upset or stress.

RANGE OF MOVEMENT
The normal measurement of the extent of movement around a specific joint or body part.

RUDE HEALTH
Vigorous good health.

SELF-LIMITING CONDITIONS
An illness or condition that will either resolve on its own or that has no long-term harmful effect on a person's health.

SOMATIC
Of the body.

SOMATIC INTELLIGENCE
The inherent ability of the body to perform tasks unconsciously, in an integrated way, involving the body, mind and emotions.

SQUAT SPLASH
See cold splash.

SUPPRESSION
The way that most medications work, they suppress the symptoms of the disease rather than dealing with the causes.

TOXAEMIA
First evolved as a concept by Dr John Tilden and published in 1926. His observations showed that most diseases are caused by an unhealthy internal state.
In his words:

Disease of the organism occurs when the waste products of normal cell metabolism cannot be expelled as quickly as they are being produced, and accumulations of potentially toxic waste are instead stored in the adjacent tissues.

Any treatment that suppresses the body's effort at elimination means that the toxins stay in the body and chronic conditions start. See Healing Crisis.

WAIST COMPRESS

See Cold Compress. The application of a cold wet cotton cloth with a woollen covering. Most often used around the waist.

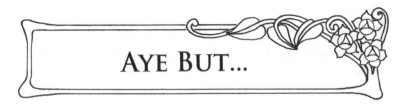

AYE BUT...

Q: So what's the difference between a Nature Cure practitioner and a Naturopath?

A: Nature Cure practitioners are also known as Naturopaths, but currently most people who practice Naturopathy also prescribe supplements as routine. We prefer to get all of the essential micronutrients, vitamins and minerals from our food. Otherwise our approaches are broadly similar.

Q: What's so wrong with supplements?

A: The body tends to use whatever comes into the system first and often this is a synthetic supplement rather than the organised and natural source in a well-balanced diet. This is one reason why we recommend that you eat organically grown foods that have been shown to have a higher percentage of naturally occurring micro-nutrients than those conventionally grown.

Q: Is it like Homeopathy?

A: No, although the initial consultations might be much the same, there are fundamental differences. In addition to a consultation the Nature Cure practitioner will also want to assess your skeletal structure and the state of your tissue, so some body work will be involved. The other big difference is that we do not prescribe any remedies. We will advise and explain but there will be no bottle or packet to take home. Instead you will learn to trust your own body's innate healing capabilities and allow them to work by understanding the steps you need to take to get back to good health naturally.

Q: Is it Herbalism?

A: No, see the answer above. Herbalists work in a similar way to orthodox doctors; in as much as they identify a problem or symptom, and prescribe a remedy to treat that symptom. They use natural herbal substances instead of mass-produced synthetic drugs. Our view is that too much emphasis and belief is put into the substance as the healer, rather than being given to our own amazing bodies.

Q: What if I already have a chronic condition?

A: It is often possible to adjust your diet and lifestyle to make your symptoms more manageable. In some cases it may even be possible to achieve a reasonable recovery, but this would require a real commitment. See Catarrhal Tendencies.

Q: Isn't telling people to keep down their fluid intake a bit counter intuitive?

A: It can certainly seem like that on first hearing, but we have many reasons for recommending limiting your fluid intake. There are times when a higher level of fluid may be needed, for instance if you are on particular medications. Keeping those highly toxic substances diluted can offer your body a better chance of being able to deal with them successfully. But, that aside, we prefer to get the bulk of our fluid intake from plant sources where they are accompanied by a fair compliment of organised minerals and vitamins. If your diet is rich in fresh vegetables, fruit and salads and low in seasoning and spices then you are unlikely to become seriously thirsty or dehydrated in the Northern Hemisphere. See 'Be Kind To Your Kidneys', 'The Healthy Human Gut' and 'What To Eat For Health' for a deeper explanation.

Q: What's is really wrong with coffee?

A: That's an interesting one. Some research has indicated that drinking coffee, with the active ingredient caffeine, can have some beneficial effects. This may be broadly true, but caffeine is a psychoactive drug and should therefore be taken in moderation. Even then, it's not so much the coffee as such, as the amount you drink, when you drink it and why you are drinking it. The odd cup of coffee, in convivial surroundings will probably do you nothing but good. Its when you feel you need to have several cups of coffee before you can function in the morning and then have several more as the day progresses 'to keep you going', that you are using caffeine as a drug. The danger here is that you become addicted, push your body too hard and risk breakdown.

Q: Why am I getting stomach upsets when I am eating a good diet?

A: There are many different reasons this could be happening. You could be eating too fast, drinking while eating, eating too much – and this is true even with good honest food – or eating in a stressful environment. Your digestive system is very sensitive to your emotional state and often it is the first part of your body to let you know that something is not right. If you have discomfort after a meal, miss the next one and have only simple fluids (not teas and coffees) for the next, then have only simple fare and in a convivial situation. If your stomach upsets persist consult a Nature Cure practitioner.

Q: You talk about growing your own vegetables, but what if I don't have a garden?

A: You can grow useful amounts of salads in pots on windowsills, or sprout seeds in glass jars. Try to get an allotment, or share one, or hassle your local authority to rent you one! Possibly you could find someone with a garden and offer to help in return for a little space to grow vegetables.

Q: What if I am on a limited income and cannot afford fresh food?

A: Think back to what folk ate between the wars. They had to make do with very basic ingredients; many of us have lost the art of cooking from scratch and need to reassess what we chose to buy. There might be a local food group were you could buy pulses and nuts in bulk and save some pennies that way. Some green groups like Zero Waste have helpful tips on their website.

Q: Why do you always give me the same answer, even though my symptoms might be different?

A: Another interesting one. It can seem like that, and often two patients at the Kingston Clinic would compare notes and find that although they had very different symptoms they had been put on the same diet and exercise regime. Nature Cure is very basic and straightforward and often advice is given to address imbalances in diet and lifestyle and it can start to sound very similar and rather familiar. As an illustration: 'Huh' said one of my cousins, 'the answer is always the same. Stop eating, put on a compress and go to bed'. And following that advice does several things in an acute condition: It gives your body a rest from digestion, some respite from work and life's stresses and allows some space for repair and rejuvenation.

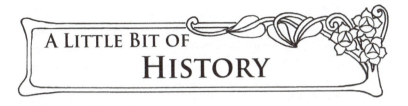

A LITTLE BIT OF HISTORY

AT THE AGE OF 17, after 18 months in the navy, James C Thomson was diagnosed with an incurable lung condition. The naval doctors delivered the news, with a hearty slap on his back, that he had only three months to live. James was so incensed by their attitude that he vowed to get better, if only to spite them. As a schoolboy he used to haunt the bookshops in Edinburgh and loved to collect books about hydrotherapy, dietetics, positive thought and actinotherapy. He thought they were very amusing and that the proponents were quacks.

But, after such a bleak prognosis, he returned home to his mother and two sisters in Edinburgh, and started to read the books again. He devised himself a daily regime and gradually his health started to improve, his mother sent him off to a cousin's farm in Perthshire to get some fresh air, healthy exercise and good honest food. With his health pretty much restored he decided to visit America where there were several different natural health movements that he wanted to learn more about.

James found himself eventually at the sanatorium of Dr Henry Lindlahr in Chicago, Illinois. He had arrived there via Bernarr MacFadden's Physical Culture centre and Kellogg's hydrotherapy sanitarium, but James hadn't felt good about what he found at Battle Creek, and didn't think their methods were right for him. Lindlahr himself had been a very ill young man, overweight and suffering from diabetes, but finding no answers from orthodox practitioners in America he travelled to Europe and sought the help of Father Kneipp. Kneipp told him that he had the 'glutton's disease' and put him on a strict diet and a course of hydrotherapy. Interestingly, Father Kneipp himself had suffered from a chronic lung condition when he was a young man, and had sought the help of Vincent Preissnitz to affect a cure; his treatment included diet, exercise, rest, sunbathing and hydrotherapy and these were to form the cornerstones of Nature Cure treatment regimes. Lindlahr made a complete recovery under Kneipp and returned to America. He went on to study at the National Medical University, adding to his knowledge of chemistry, and introduced a more scientific approach to Nature Cure. Finding a true kindred spirit, James settled in Chicago and trained in Natural Therapeutics under Lindlahr, quickly progressing to a management position in the sanatorium and proving very popular with the patients.

It was just over 100 years ago that James returned to his home country for a short holiday and to visit his mother and two sisters Eva and Agnes. To pass the time he started taking a few patients, quickly earning himself the nickname 'the Sunshine Doctor' after his recommendations for sunbathing as part of a regime towards better health. It was during this period that he was introduced to Miss Jessie Hood, a young lady suffering from an incurable heart condition. He successfully treated her and they were married in 1913. In 1914 their first child, Leslie, was born. Any plans to return to Chicago were shelved, partly due to the fact that practicing alternative medicine over in America was now becoming more difficult.

Jessie trained under James and together they practiced Nature Cure in Albany Street. After the arrival of their third child, Joyce – a sister for Leslie and Hazel, they found the house too small for a growing family as well as a growing practice. They moved, much to James's delight, to Drumsheugh Gardens, which was at that time

LIVE WELL. EAT WELL. BE WELL.

the very heart of the medical establishment. They were there for some 20 years and established the Edinburgh School of Natural Therapeutics to train practitioners. During that time Leslie studied pure science at Edinburgh University at the same time undertaking the five-year Natural Therapeutics course. Jessie also established her Free Clinic for local children, this was before the days of the NHS and many poorer families couldn't afford to pay for treatment.

There had always been a hankering to run a residential clinic; James believed that they could do so much more for their patients if they could offer accommodation as well as treatment. So in 1938, the long-time wish was fulfilled and the Kingston Clinic was opened. For some 50 years this renowned clinic was run on the south side of Edinburgh in a gothic red sandstone mansion designed by Pilkington. Surrounded by eight acres of its own grounds, including over two acres of organic kitchen garden, the clinic and extended family welcomed patients and students from all over the world.

The Clinic could accommodate around 30 patients and up to ten students, and the Edinburgh School of Natural Therapeutics was re-housed there too. The Free Clinic continued and the organic garden supplied salads and vegetables to the kitchens. No chemicals were used in the grounds; no medication was given to the patients; just support, good honest food, massage, hydrotherapy, counseling and advice about the health philosophy of Nature Cure. Students of the Edinburgh School of Natural Therapeutics graduated and set up in practice around the UK and beyond, working with this truly holistic approach. Over the years many, many patients benefitted, too often when orthodox medicine had previously let them down.

The Kingston Clinic was a truly family run business; Leslie, Hazel and Joyce got married and their spouses all worked in the clinic. Joyce's husband Alec Milne became the partner of Leslie when James died, and Hazel went south with her husband Peter LaBarre to establish another residential clinic at Blunham in Bedfordshire. Hazel was to return to Kingston when her marriage failed. There were ten healthy children born to the three families, and we all played in the grounds and eventually went our separate ways in life.

One of the legacies from the 50 years of the Kingston Clinic is a huge body of written work. A major contributor to this was the Kingston Chronicle, a periodical that the Thomson family published every couple of months. It contained comment on current topics and medical issues, gave self-help advice and offered information on different conditions for patients and it regularly featured guest writers. It was first produced in 1947 and continued until 1967. Many of the Thomson Publications monographs were first serialised in the Chronicle, and many of the resultant booklets are still available in their original format. There were published books on 'Your Heart', 'Healthy Hair', and 'Kingston Recipes'. Probably the most popular title, reprinted several times, was Jessie R Thomson's *Healthy Childhood*.

Another legacy of the Clinic was the Tait Vision Fund; this was established in 1948 and came out of the desire of a grateful patient, Adam Tait, to fund the purchase of an additional property to be run as a Nature Cure clinic and to support patients who could not afford to pay the full fees for treatment. Sadly, his family contested the will and in the end no funds were forthcoming. However, in true James C Thomson style, he set about fundraising and soon donations were flowing in from other Kingstonites. The Fund is still active today and regularly supports those on low incomes seeking Nature Cure treatment. It also supports activities to promote Nature Cure.

Nature Cure is still alive and well, although the old school have since retired or passed away. There is a new distance learning course being run, which is currently based in York, new books coming out, and interactive websites. Things come and go, Nature Cure has always been there, but it is poised ready for a fresh blossoming of interest.

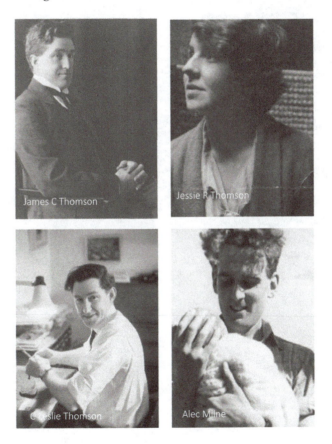

James C Thomson

Jessie R Thomson

C Leslie Thomson

Alec Milne

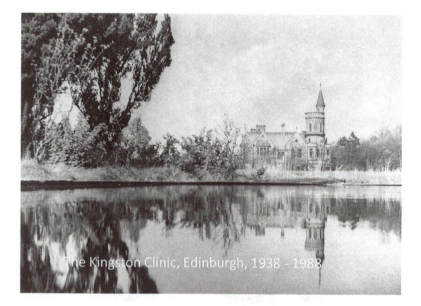

The Kingston Clinic, Edinburgh, 1938 - 1988

BIBLIOGRAPHY

The Living Soil. Balfour, Lady Eve. 1975

The Sleep Solution. Ball, Nigel and Hough, Nick. 1998

Earth Matters. Bargett, Richard D. 2015

Games People Play. Berne, Dr Eric. 1987

Missing Microbes. Blaser, Dr Martin. 2014

What to Eat. Blythman, Joanna. 2009

Right Relationships. Brown, Peter G and Garver, Geoffrey. 2009

The Feminization of Nature. Cadbury, Deborah. 1998

The Silent Spring. Carson, Rachel. 1962

On Men, Masculinity in Crisis. Clare, Professor Anthony. 1991

How to Stop Your Doctor Killing You. Coleman, Vernon. 2003

The Art of Happiness, A Handbook for Living. Dalai Lama. 1999

Nutritional Medicine. Davies, Stewart and Stanway. 1987

The Selfish Gene. Dawkins, Richard. 2006

The Healing Power of Illness. Thirwald Deflethsen and Ruediger Dahike.
    1999

Fit For Life. Diamond, Harvey. 1989

Gut. Enders, Giulia. 2014

The Art of Loving. Fromm, Erich. 1995

Bad Pharma. Goldacre, Ben. 2013

Emotional Intelligence. Goleman, Daniel. 1996

Deadly Medicines and Organised Crime. Gotzsche, Peter. 2013

Biotechnology Unzipped. Grace, Eric S. 2006

Human Givens. Griffin, Joe and Tyrell, Ivan. 2013

Trust Me (I'm Still a Doctor). Hammond, Dr Phil. 2009

I'm OK, You're OK. Harris, Thomas A. 1995 and 2012

The Killing of the Countryside. Harvey, Graham. 1997

The Great Food Gamble. Humphrys, John. 2002

Fringe Medicine. Inglis, Brian. 1964

Passage to Power. Kenton, Lesley. 1998

Middle Aged Rebel. Lambley, Peter. 1995

Natural Therapeutics. Lindlahr, Dr Henry. 2004

It Ain't Necessarily So, The Dream of the Human Genome. Lewontin, Richard. 2000

Chemical Children. Mansfield, Peter and Munro, Jean. 1987

Nature Cure. Maybe, Richard. 2005

The Patient Paradox. McCartney, Dr Margaret. 2012

Soil & Soul. McIntosh, Alastair. 2004

What Doctors Don't Tell You. McTaggart, Lynne. 2005

Depression, How to Survive it. Milligan, Spike and Clare, Professor Anthony. 1994

Women Who Love Too Much. Norwood, Robin. 2004

Menopause Without Medicine. Ojeda, Linda. 1998

Earth in Mind. Orr, David W. 1994

Why Men Don't Listen & Women Can't Read Maps. Pease, Allan and Barbara. 2001

Molecules of Emotion. Pert, Dr Candace. 1997

The Chimp Paradox. Peters, Professor Steve. 2014

In Defence of Food. Pollen, Michael. 2008

A Natural Profession. Power, Richenda. 2016

Back in Ten Minutes. Rintoul, Dr Mary and West, Bernard. 1995

Don't Worry – It's Safe to Eat. Rowell, Andrew. 2003

The Ultimate Heresy. Seymour, John. 1999

Families and How to Survive Them. Skynner, Robin and Cleese, John. 1989

How to Survive Without Psychotherapy. Small, David. 1998

An Introduction to Nature Cure. Thomson, James and Jessie. 1916

The Power of Now. Tolle, Eckhart. 2001

Mindfulness. Williams, Mark and Penman, Danny. 2011

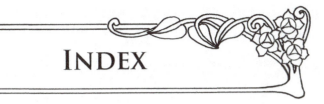

INDEX

LIVE WELL. EAT WELL. BE WELL.

THE INCORPORATED SOCIETY
OF REGISTERED NATUROPATHS

This logo represents a fresh flowering of Nature Cure; we felt it was time for a new logo to represent Nature Cure and the long-established Incorporated Society of Registered Naturopaths as it moves into its second century.

THE PETALS

The original logo (or icon) was based on a square sitting on the ancient conventional symbols for Earth, Air, Fire and Water. The new logo has five petals to represent the five senses: Touch, Taste, Smell, Hearing and Sight. The colours in the logo also represent those older established elements.

THE CIRCLE

The circle in blue represents the circle of consciousness, as it sits within the petals but is not bound by them. It also represents water; essential to health and life. It is also our blue planet, our earth that we live and depend upon.

THE TRIANGLE

The triangle represents creative thought but also the stability of the trinity. The three leaf-shaped arms of the triangle also contain the words: Spiritual & Emotional, Science & Philosophy and Mental & Physical. The four concepts sit above the ways that we study them. These three foundation stones in turn surround a Spiral of Intuition. These concepts all contribute to make the whole human being. If any one of them dominates or is missing, the individual becomes unbalanced.

The single flower is the individual; every part of the flower continuously affects all other parts. No one part is more important

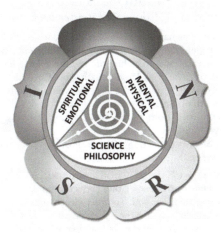

than any other and each part contributes to the mental, physical and emotional balance of the individual. The petals reach out to the external world and take in the healing power of the sun, fresh air, clean water, well-tended earth and warming fire.

www.naturecuresociety.co.uk

The illustration at the beginning of each of the chapters is based on the flower symbol.

Luath Press Limited
committed to publishing well written books worth reading

LUATH PRESS takes its name from Robert Burns, whose little collie Luath (*Gael.*, swift or nimble) tripped up Jean Armour at a wedding and gave him the chance to speak to the woman who was to be his wife and the abiding love of his life. Burns called one of 'The Twa Dogs' Luath after Cuchullin's hunting dog in Ossian's *Fingal*. Luath Press was established in 1981 in the heart of Burns country, and now resides a few steps up the road from Burns' first lodgings on Edinburgh's Royal Mile. Luath offers you distinctive writing with a hint of unexpected pleasures.

Most bookshops in the UK, the US, Canada, Australia, New Zealand and parts of Europe either carry our books in stock or can order them for you. To order direct from us, please send a £sterling cheque, postal order, international money order or your credit card details (number, address of cardholder and expiry date) to us at the address below. Please add post and packing as follows: UK – £1.00 per delivery address; overseas surface mail – £2.50 per delivery address; overseas airmail – £3.50 for the first book to each delivery address, plus £1.00 for each additional book by airmail to the same address. If your order is a gift, we will happily enclose your card or message at no extra charge.

Luath Press Limited
543/2 Castlehill
The Royal Mile
Edinburgh EH1 2ND
Scotland
Telephone: 0131 225 4326 (24 hours)
email: sales@luath.co.uk
Website: www.luath.co.uk